HOMEOPATHIC CELL SALT REMEDIES

HEALING WITH NATURE'S 12 MINERAL COMPOUNDS

D1295175

NIGEY LENNON
LIONEL ROLFE

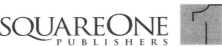

SQUAREONE
PUBLISHERS

The information and advice contained in this book are based upon the research, the interviews, and the personal experiences of the authors. They are not intended as a substitute for consulting with a health care professional. The publisher and authors are not responsible for any adverse effects or consequences resulting from the use of any of the suggestions, preparations, or procedures discussed in this book. All matters pertaining to your physical health should be supervised by a health care professional. It is a sign of wisdom, not cowardice, to seek a second or third opinion.

COVER DESIGNER: Jeannie Tudor
IN-HOUSE EDITOR: Rudy Shur
TYPESETTER: Gary A. Rosenberg

Square One Publishers

115 Herricks Road
Garden City Park, N.Y. 11040
(516) 535-2010 • (877) 900-BOOK
www.squareonepublishers.com

Library of Congress Cataloging-in-Publication Data
Lennon, Nigey, 1954–
    Homeopathic cell salt remedies : healing with nature's twelve mineral compounds / Nigey Lennon and Lionel Rolfe.
        p. cm.
    Includes index.
    ISBN 0-7570-0250-1 (pbk.)
    1. Medicine, Biochemic. 2. Salts—Therapeutic use.
3. Schüssler, Wilhelm Heinrich, 1821–1898. 4. Homeopathy.
I. Rolfe, Lionel, 1942– II. Title.
RZ412.L46   2004
615.2—dc22
                                                          2004008317

Copyright © 2004 by Nigey Lennon and Lionel Rolfe

Printed in the United States of America

10   9   8   7

Contents

Introduction

B efore his death, Dr. Linus Pauling, winner of two Nobel Prizes for chemistry and world peace, predicted that the greatest advances in the twenty-first century would be in medicine, biochemistry, and molecular biology. He theorized that the motion of atoms and the way in which this motion relates to health and disease would become far better understood as the century progressed.

Dr. Pauling believed that the future of medicine would not be in the use of medical treatments for particular illnesses, but rather that the trend would be toward the development of medicines for each individual person—medicines which, like a fingerprint, would reflect an individual's unique physical attributes, and would specifically assist each person in maintaining optimal health. This advanced concept is, surprisingly, remarkably similar to the theory of a school of medicine that originated in Germany more than two centuries ago. It is known as homeopathic medicine.

Dr. Wilhelm Heinrich Schuessler (1821–1898) was born in Oldenburg, Germany. He almost single-handedly revolutionized homeopathic medicine in the mid-nineteenth century. Dr. Schuessler, a homeopathic physician, felt that the 2,000 or so homeopathic remedies used in his day could be simplified. Determining that the active ingredients in this vast array of remedies were their mineral constituents, he worked in his laboratory to isolate the mineral components, which ultimately resulted in twelve individual remedies. These became known as the Schuessler cell salts.

Today, much of the homeopathic cell salt-based medicine practiced throughout the world is founded on Dr. Schuessler's work. Since the twentieth century, homeopathy has enjoyed widespread popularity in Germany, France, parts of Latin America, Mexico, and India. The cell salts are widely used in Great Britain (Queen Elizabeth's royal physician is a homeopathic practitioner). In Russia, large homeopathic clinics and hospitals are operating in major population centers.

In the United States, homeopathy and the cell salt system have primarily been kept alive through the efforts of laymen rather than by medical professionals. Conventional medical doctors here are relatively unfamiliar with homeopathy, even though it was in a homeopathic hospital in New York that x-rays were first used in the fight against cancer.

Now, however, as public interest in self-care and natural remedies grows by leaps and bounds in the United States, the awareness of homeopathy has become increasingly widespread. Many people are discovering for themselves that cell salts can keep them well, especially when used as part of an overall approach to good health. The remedies themselves are easily obtainable, in retail outlets as well as online and by mail order.

Cell salts can have many extremely positive effects on your health. Although you take a particular remedy based on your symptoms, these medicines produce results not by simply eliminating the symptoms, but by correcting the imbalances that have caused the symptoms in the first place. Because of this, you will find that these remedies can cure far more than the symptoms for which you may have originally taken them. Furthermore, the more you involve yourself in maintaining your own health, including learning about and using cell salts, the more you will benefit.

The purpose of this book is to give an overview of the many benefits of the twelve cell salts, and to serve as a guide to their best uses in promoting and maintaining wellness. It goes without saying that the cell salts should be used for the sort of health problems that call for self-diagnosis, self-treatment, and self-medication. If you have any doubt about the seriousness of a particular ailment, you should consult a physician. It is advisable, as well, to consider an initial consultation with a homeopathic practitioner. He or she will take a detailed health history and will be able to answer any questions you may have about the use of the remedies in your particular situation. This is not absolutely necessary, but it can prove a valuable first step before beginning any cell salt program.

The twelve Schuessler cell salts have the advantage of being simple enough for almost anyone to use, while at the same time they are extremely powerful in fighting ailments and promoting health and wellness. Once you understand the different cell salts and how to use them to treat specific problems, you can take charge of your own health and begin to experience increased vitality and well-being. To your health and self-knowledge!

Part I

An Introduction to Cell Salts

1.

A History of Cell Salts

Dr. Hahnemann and the Birth of Homeopathy

For well over a century, the twelve cell salt remedies have been keeping people fit and healthy. To understand how and why they work, it is necessary to take a closer look at homeopathy, the medical philosophy from which the cell salts evolved.

In the eighteenth century, German physician and scientist Samuel Hahnemann (1755–1843) developed a medical concept which became known as homeopathy: the prefix *homo*, in Greek, means "same." After conducting extensive research with thousands of botanical medicines, Dr. Hahnemann evolved the hypothesis that "like cures like"; his research indicated that the same substance which caused the symptoms of a particular disease in a healthy patient often resulted in curing those *same* symptoms when someone was ill. Vaccinations are an example of this theory in action. When a minute amount of a pathogen is introduced into the body, the immune system identifies that pathogen and arms itself against infection.

Another revolutionary discovery made by Hahnemann was that the very smallest dosage of a particular remedy—less than one part per million—was more effective than the large doses commonly given. In his day, large quantities of medicinal substances were routinely dispensed to patients. Hahnemann's theory, that minute quantities of a substance could directly penetrate the tissues and enable an individual to restore healthy bodily processes on a cell-by-cell basis, was far ahead of its time, as vaccinations only came into general use in the mid-nineteenth century.

In *An Introduction to the Principles and Practice of Homeopathy,*
Charles E. Wheeler, MD, consulting physician to the London
Homeopathic Hospital and former president of the British Home-
opathic Society, explains that:

> the success of vaccine therapy comes to strengthen the pos-
> sibility that 'like' may be a remedy for 'like,' for if it is not
> homeopathy to make remedies for diseases out of the agents
> which are held to be the causes of these diseases it is difficult
> to find a better word. . . . Vaccine therapy does not prove the
> truth of homeopathy, but does it not make it less paradoxical
> and incite to independent research?

These two ideas—like curing like, and the minimum dose—
became the cornerstone of homeopathic medicine. It also led to
a sharp division between the two factions of medical practice,
homeopaths and *allopaths* (non-homeopathic doctors). Historical-
ly, homeopathy represented a major step forward in both medical
theory and practice. As late as the nineteenth century it was common practice for allopathic physicians to routinely administer
toxic drugs in large quantities or to apply parasitic leeches to
"purify" the patient's blood. Physicians' ignorance of medical
hygiene also often resulted in spreading infection from patient to
patient when they failed to wash their hands.

With its holistic focus, homeopathy shifted the paradigm
away from external medical modalities and gross remedies, and
toward the notion that each patient was a unique individual who
required individual diagnosis and a remedy specific to his or her
case. As we shall see, this philosophy not only predated many
modern medical discoveries, it also empowered patients to take
more responsibility for their own treatment.

Hahnemann's work in homeopathic medicine led to the formation of several homeopathic institutes in his native Germany.
Subsequently, homeopathy became a well accepted medical practice in that country, and by the mid-nineteenth century it had
spread to many other countries in Europe, as well as started gaining widespread acceptance in the United States.

The Contribution of Dr. Schuessler

A half-century after Dr. Hahnemann's revolutionary discoveries, Wilhelm H. Schuessler was practicing homeopathic medicine in the village of Oldenburg, Germany. A brilliant man, Dr. Schuessler had mastered Greek, Latin, and Sanskrit as well as English, Italian, and Spanish, and had read widely in the medical literature of those languages. From almost the beginning of his career, he had worked to simplify the more than 2,000 remedies of the homeopathic materia medica (repertory of medicines).

Dr. Schuessler was influenced by the pioneering work of Dr. Rudolph Virchow, the father of modern pathology. Dr. Virchow theorized that the disturbances thought of as diseases are actually signs of change in cell metabolism. Based on this idea, Dr. Schuessler became further convinced that the active ingredients in the most successful homeopathic remedies were inorganic. His research led him to conclude that when the human cell is reduced to ashes, there are only twelve minerals left.

Taking the theory of the minimum dose into account, Dr. Schuessler reasoned that a lack of these minerals in a living organism will keep organic materials from entering the cells, which in turn prohibits the cells from performing their natural functions. Thus, he suggested that these twelve minerals be taken in homeopathic doses in order to regulate individual cell function.

How the Twelve Cell Salts Work to Restore Health

Dr. Schuessler's system of twelve cell salts condenses the thousands of medicines found in the homeopathic materia medica into twelve basic remedies, and submits that these twelve remedies can do most of the things that the thousands of others can do. There are homeopathic practitioners who dispute the idea that these twelve remedies can replace the entire materia medica. However, because of their simplicity and accessibility, laymen can easily learn how to use them effectively for many health problems.

Dr. Schuessler believed that the active ingredients in homeopathic remedies are the inorganic minerals that affect cell metabolism. For example, one of the most famous homeopathic botanical remedies is *pulsatilla,* which is obtained from the coneflower (*pulsatilla*). Even before Dr. Schuessler, homeopathic doctors understood that the active ingredient in *pulsatilla* was silica—a mineral. In homeopathic practice, the cell salt remedy silica is often viewed as a refinement of the botanical remedy *pulsatilla,* to be routinely given in cases where *pulsatilla* has failed to provide relief.

Cell salts are necessary when the cells are lacking in certain nutrients, creating a cellular imbalance. In a very real sense, when you take a cell salt remedy, you are supplying a micro-nutrient that enables your body to rebuild itself on the cellular level.

The twelve Schuessler cell salts, like all homeopathic remedies, are prepared in minute doses. The smaller the active ingredient, the easier it is for it to enter the cells and the more powerful the effect it has on cellular function. Manufacturing of the salts begins with a careful determination of the quality of the minerals. Only the best grade of minerals is used from natural sources.

In the first step of the manufacturing process, the minerals are ground by hand—a process which takes at least 200 hours. The finer the particles of the minerals and the higher the potency being manufactured, the longer the grinding takes. After the mineral has been ground to a fine powder in the laboratory, which is hermetically sealed to prevent any dust from escaping, the powder is transferred to an electrically driven mortar and pestle. The potency of the cell salt is determined by the length of time it is ground in the mortar and pestle.

Eventually, the active ingredient is vaporized, and at that point the air in the laboratory is full of the mineral. The operator who removes the vaporized mineral substance from the mortar and pestle must wear a mask, because the vapor has incredible powers of penetration. The final tablets are made up of the mineral and milk sugar.

In the Schuessler dosages, far less than one part per million of the mineral is present in the cell salt tablet. The active mineral ingredient is said to be *triturated*—ground extremely finely. In Chapter 3 we will describe the various dosages of the various cell salt tablets.

Health on a Cellular Level

Each individual cell of your body is a marvelous organism that normally selects or rejects substances to maintain health. When disease or irritation is present, the cell loses this ability to regulate its processes. Thus, weakened cells must receive the mineral they need in triturated form. Bypassing the digestive system is necessary to overcome the cell's inability to absorb nutrients from the digestive system.

It might seem strange to think of health as being determined by such microscopic processes, but this is definitely the case. One biochemist made a fascinating microscopic film showing how a small amount of poison (one part in one million) quickly went to work destroying cells. Seeing this demonstrated so graphically, it is easy to understand how damaging pollutants can be in our air, food, and water.

Also, medical research has shown that disease begins at the cellular level. For instance, healthy cells require two mutations to become cancerous. If we understand how to maintain healthy cell function, it will ultimately be possible to prevent these mutations from occurring. Taking cell salts will not necessarily prevent cancer, of course, but taking charge of your health from the inside out—as you do when you learn which cell salt works best to combat a particular ailment—is certainly good insurance in keeping yourself healthy.

As is made clear with each new scientific discovery, health is a subtle process. Your input into the process is critical; you have to take the initiative if you want to stay healthy. You need to be concerned not only with good nutrition, but also with such issues as pollution, the chemicals in the foods you eat, and everything that enters your body. Dr. Schuessler's cell salts are most effective as part of this holistic approach to wellness—taking as much care as you can of your whole body and its environment. In this way, the cell salts can be of great assistance by helping you regulate and balance your biochemical processes at the cellular level.

Perhaps the most positive aspect of the cell salts is that they can be self-administered. With little more than this book and a few dollars for the inexpensive remedies (available by mail, online, and at many natural foods stores), you can effectively treat many of your illnesses, and in the process experience an overall sense of health and vitality that you may never have felt before.

There is no mystery surrounding cell salts and their many benefits. If you suffer from the common cold, for instance, when you take the appropriate cell salt remedy you will find the relief that is promised (but never delivered) by widely advertised over-the-counter medicines. It is important to realize that *you cannot harm yourself with cell salts*. Even if your body has no need of a particular cell salt you may be taking, no damage will be done.

Each cell salt, as you will see, performs a specific function in the body's vital processes, and all of these functions and process-es are interrelated. Homeopathic medicine emphasizes the individuality of each person. Each person will have characteristic symptoms that spell out his or her need for particular remedies.

How a Homeopathic Practitioner Can Help You

While homeopathy is especially useful in matters of self-diagno-sis and self-prescription, there are instances when professional evaluation, judgment, and prescription are indicated. If you have any doubts about the seriousness of an ailment, or if you have been taking a particular cell salt or other remedy for an extended period without obtaining relief, you should consult a physician.

Even if you do not think you have a serious health problem, a consultation with a homeopathic practitioner can provide you with much useful information. A homeopathic practitioner will take a detailed medical history, which, as you will see, can be extremely helpful in understanding which remedies you might need. He or she can also advise you about appropriate remedies.

However, the advantage of the Schuessler cell salts is that any-one with a little basic information can identify and treat a whole host of everyday ailments, and that is what this book will help you do. In the next chapter, we will start by examining the twelve individual cell salts, and gaining an understanding of the role each plays in the body's processes.

2.

The Twelve Cell Salts

As we have discussed, Dr. Schuessler's homeopathic remedies are comprised of twelve cell salts. In order to function properly, our bodies' cells require these cell salts or minerals. By providing a homeopathic dose of one or more of these minerals, the body can restore health first on a cellular level and then on a systemic level.

In the following summaries, the cell salts are referred to by their full general names (e.g. calcium fluoride), with their older homeopathic short-hand names in parentheses (*calc. fluor.*). Some cell salt manufacturers market cell salts under the general name, while others stick to the homeopathic designation.

Calcium Fluoride (*Calc. fluor.*)
A NATURAL PRODUCER OF SUPPLENESS AND ELASTICITY

Calcium fluoride (*calc. fluor.*) is a constituent of the surfaces of bones and the enamel of teeth. It is also a prime ingredient in elastic fibers in the body. It is a chemical union of lime and fluoric acid. This bond produces a remedy with healing powers greater than either of the constituents alone.

Calcium fluoride is useful in treating many ailments of the bones and teeth. Many experts blame the unusual amount of dental and interstitial (gum) problems seen in Americans not only on poor diet, but also on a lack of calcium. There is, of course, calcium in milk and milk products, but there are indications that the pasteurization process adversely affects calcium. People with sensitive teeth or gums may require calcium fluoride.

As a prime ingredient in connective tissues in the body, calcium fluoride is often of importance in treating diseases of the skin and the blood vessels. Hemorrhoids and varicose veins often respond well to treatment with this cell salt.

People with heart trouble can find a great deal of relief with calcium fluoride. Of course, heart problems can be very serious, so it is not advisable to attempt self-treatment in such cases. But calcium fluoride can be a powerful ally in your overall treatment plan.

Calcium fluoride is sometimes recommended to overweight people, to be taken an hour before each meal in alternation with calcium phosphate. The idea is that these two cell salts will aid in the assimilation of starches and fat in the meals. Cutting down on these items in the diet is also helpful in weight loss, of course.

Calcium Phosphate (*Calc. phos.*)

THE REGULATOR OF HEALTHY CELLULAR ACTIVITY

Phosphate of lime, or calcium phosphate (*calc. phos.*), is one of the major cell salt remedies. It operates by promoting healthy cellular activity. As a main constituent of all the cells and fluids in the body, it plays a major role in the health of the muscular, skeletal, excretory, and lymphatic systems.

It is interesting to note that calcium phosphate is a main ingredient in the most productive soils; the gardener who is unfamiliar with calcium phosphate as a soil additive is a poor gardener indeed. Not surprisingly, it is one of the first cell salts to take if you are feeling generally run-down, as well as the primary remedy for children who are not growing or developing properly.

This cell salt tends to intensify the action of other cell salts in promoting healthy cellular function and restoring tone to weakened organs and tissues, so it is often taken in conjunction with many other cell salts. Calcium phosphate is known for its restorative powers after acute diseases and infections. It can be very helpful for people who catch colds easily. It is useful for many disorders of the reproductive organs, especially in women.

Calcium Sulphate (*Calc. sulph.*)
HEALER AND PURIFIER OF THE SKIN AND EXTERNAL TISSUES

Calcium sulphate (*calc. sulph.*) has been in medical use for years in making casts. Eggshells are made of this material, and farmers use it in soil to improve the color of grapes. But it was homeopathic practitioners who first recognized its medical value when taken internally. Because calcium sulphate will hold water but tends to resist acid, some practitioners believe that it acts as a protecting influence against acidic fluids.

It is useful in protecting the stomach walls as well as the eyeballs, nasal passages, mouth, throat, bladder, and any other organs that need protection against moisture. Since the skin can suffer from many kinds of external wounds and damage, it is good to know that you can look to calcium sulphate as a remedy for these.

It is a great healer of wounds and skin ailments. It works in conjunction with silica (see page 18) to heal wounds that are discharging pus and to promote healing. Calcium sulphate can also be useful in treating some types of rheumatism, since it is an important element in the body's connective tissues.

Ferrum Phosphate (*Ferrum phos.*)
POWERFUL OXYGENATOR

Ferrum phosphate (*ferrum phos.*) is a powerful oxygenator, carrying oxygen throughout the bloodstream and strengthening the walls of the blood vessels, especially in the arteries. Because oxygen-rich blood is essential to vital health, ferrum phosphate is critical in ailments characterized by congestion, inflammation, fever, or rapid pulse.

Ferrum phosphate makes iron available to the cells in minute doses, thus bypassing the side effects (such as mineral buildup or constipation) of iron taken in large amounts. Naturally, it is the first cell salt remedy to consider in cases of anemia. Since it is a blood tonic, purifying the blood and helping to regulate immune function, in many instances taking it regularly will result in improved overall health and energy.

Magnesium Phosphate (*Mag. phos.*)
ANTI-SPASMODIC REMEDY

Magnesium phosphate (*mag. phos.*) is one of the most remarkable cell salt remedies. While it is very powerful when used alone, it is also closely allied with the other two phosphate cell salts—calcium phosphate and potassium phosphate. In combination, the phosphates are an excellent tonic for the nerves. It is through our nerves that we experience the sensation of pain, so the phosphates, and magnesium phosphate specifically, can be very helpful in pain relief.

Potassium phosphate operates on the gray nerve fibers, and magnesium phosphate on the white ones. The two are closely connected, and if there is a disturbance of the molecules of the gray fibers, there will almost inevitably also be a disturbance of the white fibers as well. Many cell salt practitioners, therefore, do not recommend taking one of the phosphate remedies without also including the other two.

Magnesium is quite plentiful in the body; it is a "trace" element, and is exceeded in quantity only by calcium, potassium, and sodium. Magnesium is a factor in helping the blood remain alkaline, and it works in conjunction with phosphorous in rebuilding the nerves. It also helps harden dental enamel. The metabolism of glucose in the muscles depends on a correct magnesium balance. Magnesium phosphate is needed by the brain, heart, and muscles to relax. Thus, it is helpful in cases of cramping, muscle spasm, and muscle tightness.

Potassium Chloride (*Kali mur.*)
SUBTLE-ACTING, BUT PROFOUND

Potassium chloride (*kali mur.*) is a subtle-acting cell salt and can sometimes be overshadowed by the more dramatic remedies such as ferrum phosphate or sodium chloride. Nevertheless, potassium chloride is an important constituent of the muscles, nerve cells, and brain cells. In fact, brain cells cannot form without this cell salt. From Dr. Schuessler's time to the present, homeopathic practitioners have believed that potassium chloride is the cell salt responsible for building fibrin, the protein fiber that is an essential part of the formation of blood clots.

In many ways, potassium chloride resembles potassium sulphate and is indicated in many of the same ailments. It is most helpful in treating chronic ailments, especially where severe inflammation is involved. It can help destroy bacterial waste products when the body is fighting off a fever or infection. It should be taken after the fever has broken and the body must begin the process of convalescence and rebuilding its health. Potassium chloride retards the body's secretion mechanism and can be useful in cases of discharge or excess clotting. It acts as a blood thinner, and can help restore normal blood flow through the arteries.

Potassium chloride should be taken routinely, along with ferrum phosphate, for colds and other catarrhal conditions. It is also effective, along with calcium sulphate, for certain kinds of rheumatism. Applied externally, potassium chloride is useful in controlling blistering when it is used on burns and scalds.

Potassium Phosphate (*Kali phos.*)

SOOTHER OF JANGLED NERVES

Potassium phosphate (*kali phos.*) is the most important of the three potassium cell salt remedies. Homeopathic practitioners worldwide rely on it as a safe and effective tranquilizer. For the biochemical preparation of potassium phosphate, potassium is mixed with phosphoric acid until the solution is slightly alkaline (as opposed to acid). Phosphoric acid is vital to brain chemistry because it combines with other substances and becomes part of the "gray matter" of the brain. Thus, potassium phosphate has been found to help people suffering from psychological problems such as depression, anxiety, and irritability. It helps cure headaches and restores healthful sleep patterns. This remedy is often prescribed for memory loss and dementia associated with the aging process.

Potassium phosphate operates as a "detergent" in the large intestine and alimentary canal. It is also vital to the action of the heart. Some researchers believe that the key to preventing cancer is to understand the chemical changes effected on the cells by potassium. Further research will undoubtedly clarify the connection between specific potassium levels and cellular health and will perhaps result in finding ways to utilize this most important substance in the treatment of cancer.

Potassium Sulphate (*Kali sulph.*)

CELLULAR BUILDING BLOCK

Potassium sulphate (*kali sulph.*) works together with ferrum phosphate to help carry oxygen throughout the bloodstream and into the cells. While ferrum phosphate is said to regulate the "external breathing" of cells in the exchange of gases, potassium sulphate is said to regulate the "internal breathing." Both cell salts act in concert in transporting oxygen, although potassium sulphate is believed to be able to carry oxygen in cases where ferrum phosphate cannot.

Potassium sulphate's main duty is to build new cells when the old ones have been damaged or killed due to disease. This remedy is nearly always suggested for skin problems, often in combination with other remedies.

This cell salt is often effective in treating asthma, especially bronchial asthma. It has been successful in helping people recover their senses of taste and smell when they have been suffering from nose and throat infections.

Silica (*Silica*)

REMARKABLE CELLULAR CLEANSER

Silica is one of the most abundant of the earth's solid components. It comes from rocks worn down into pebbles and then further reduced to dust by the action of wind and rain. The resulting dust becomes "grit," and is a major supportive element in the connective tissues of both plant and animal cells.

Silica literally provides "grit" in the cellular membrane and the body's connective tissues. It is a powerful cleanser and eliminator of toxins; in fact, in the pre-antibiotic days of the previous century it was sometimes known as the "homeopathic surgeon" because of its dramatic ability to assist the body in throwing off toxins and curing infections.

This cell salt is effective in causing boils and abscesses to throw off pus. It is a tonic for hair and skin, which are continuously sloughing off cells and benefit greatly from silica's strengthening properties.

Silica also relieves swelling and heat in joints and has been used successfully to dissolve the urate deposits of arthritis and gout. In cases of asthma complicated by heavy mucus on the chest, silica can significantly reduce the inflammation and restore normal breathing.

Sodium Chloride (*Natrum mur.*)
PRE-EMINENT HEADACHE REMEDY

Although it is one of the most powerful cell salts, and often acts with remarkable speed in cases of serious illness, sodium chloride (*natrum mur.*) is probably best known as the pre-eminent remedy for headaches.

Sodium chloride is present in high concentration in bodily fluids. Its chief task is the creation and stabilization of osmotic pressure, regulating the passage of fluids. The process of osmosis is crucial within the body, since without it, the cells would be unable to receive the nutrients they require, nor would they be able to conduct many biochemical processes necessitating the exchange of fluids. As a critical factor in promoting osmosis, sodium chloride is an important cell salt remedy.

This cell salt's effectiveness in relieving headaches is widely discussed in homeopathic studies. The primary cause of headaches stems from changes in blood flow. Homeopathic practitioners theorize that sodium chloride works to stabilize the blood flow to the brain, thereby reducing the severity of headaches and often eliminating them entirely.

Since it regulates the passage of fluids through the cells, sodium chloride can also be effective in reducing hypertension (high blood pressure).

Sodium Phosphate (*Natrum phos.*)

THE BIOCHEMICAL ANTACID

Sodium phosphate (*natrum phos.*) has often been called the "biochemical antacid." It is found in the blood, muscles, nerves, and brain cells, where its role is to aid in the decomposition of lactic acid and the emulsification of fatty acids. In many ailments, the common causative factor is acidity of the blood. Sodium phosphate helps reduce this acidity, and thus is helpful in ailments such as gout, back pain, muscle aches, and indigestion.

It can also be effective in some cases of rheumatism, often used in conjunction with ferrum phosphate. Phosphate never occurs in a free state; it is always found in combination with other phosphates. In combination, the four phosphate remedies are used as a standard cell salt nerve tonic.

Sodium Sulphate (*Natrum sulph.*)

REMEDY FOR ASTHMA

While sodium chloride attracts water *to* the body's tissues, sodium sulphate (*natrum sulph.*) regulates the carrying away of fluids from the cells. This makes sodium sulphate a remedy for many ailments which are aggravated or caused by dampness, including asthma. Sodium sulphate has been shown to attract twice its bulk in water-containing waste products and then remove this waste from the bloodstream. It is also known to speed healing in the mucous membranes. This cell salt has been found to act as a "sensor," assisting the cells in discerning both harmful and beneficial substances in the fluid surrounding the cells.

Sodium sulphate has been successful in treating diabetes, and in fact it can play an enormous role in eliminating many digestive problems. Homeopathic medical literature records that it can be helpful in regulating liver function, and therefore may be useful in cases of hepatitis.

While the names of these cell salts may be a little off-putting, the point to remember is that these minerals provide the basic structure and means for all life on our planet to exist. You will find that the more you use these remedies and say their names, the more familiar with these cell salts you will become. There was a time in the past when the term "antibiotic" sounded strange. Today, however, its overuse is all-too-familiar.

Now that you are better acquainted with the names and functions of Dr. Schuessler's twelve cell salts, let's learn how they can best be used.

3.

How to Use Cell Salts

Using Cell Salts to Treat Specific Problems

As you have seen in the previous chapter, each cell salt plays a specific role in the body's cellular processes. Once you understand the basic job each cell salt performs within the body, you will begin to understand which remedy to turn to when you want to treat a particular health concern. In Part II of this book, you will find listings of particular ailments along with the corresponding cell salt remedy or remedies best used to treat them.

It is important to remember that cell salts do not work in a superficial manner. You can expect them to balance and regulate many biochemical, physiological, and neurological functions; that is what they have been proven to do in more than a hundred years of applied research. When you use the exact remedy you need for a particular ailment, you will often experience instantaneous and permanent relief, because you have pinpointed the root cause of the ailment.

However, you will find that sometimes cell salts take longer to produce noticeable results. This is because it is the nature of some of the remedies to work slowly and profoundly, especially in cases of longstanding or systemic ailments. Taken in minute doses, cell salts exercise their powerful functions to repair and maintain your body's health at the cellular level. In the long run, they will help you feel better and stay healthy. But especially at first, you need to be patient while waiting for your body to respond to and assimilate the cell salt or salts you have taken, and then to begin functioning normally again.

Recognizing Your "Constitutional Remedy"

Human beings are individuals, and each of us has a different genetic and environmentally influenced set of physical capacities, immune functions, and tendencies to disease. Of course, our bodies operate in the same basic fashion as those of all our other fellow human beings. However, homeopathic medicine considers each person as an individual, especially when it comes to recognizing certain physical patterns and understanding which remedy may be required to treat a specific ailment.

In homeopathic medicine, very close attention is paid to the patient's previous medical history, past and present illnesses, metabolism, emotional makeup, and specific reactions to physical and mental factors. More than 200 years of research by homeopathic practitioners has indicated that the need for a particular remedy is clearly indicated by a unique and recognizable pattern of physical and mental factors.

You need to begin your own investigation of cell salts to discover which of the twelve remedies is your own specific *constitutional remedy*. Study the descriptions of the symptoms of particular ailments described in this book, and the corresponding cell salt remedy or remedies suggested to treat them. You will find yourself dismissing certain cell salts because you do not have the symptoms they treat. In some cases, you may have some of the symptoms but not all of them. Once you are familiar with each of the twelve cell salts and the particular roles they play in maintaining health, you will see which are right for you.

It is likely that as you study ailments and corresponding cell salts, you will recognize in yourself a specific, recurrent pattern of physical and mental factors that point to a particular remedy. This cell salt is described by homeopathic practitioners as your constitutional remedy. Once identified, it should be taken regularly, either by itself or in combination with other cell salts you may need to treat a specific ailment. Even if your constitutional remedy may not be indicated for a current health problem, you should take it regularly to maintain overall health and to support other cell salts in combating a particular ailment.

As you read this book, you will also begin to recognize some of the patterns that indicate a need for cell salts in various combinations. The phosphates, chlorides, and sulphates all work together within the cells to promote and maintain health, and should be taken together in certain instances. Consult the Simplified Remedy Guide found on page 31 for more information.

See Part II for more information on *acute* and *chronic* ailments and dosages. You will take cell salts less frequently and/or in smaller doses if you have had an illness for a long period (chronic) or in more frequent/larger doses if you are experiencing sudden, intense symptoms (acute).

How to Take Cell Salts

Cell salts are available in several different forms. The most common is a tiny tablet, which is placed under the tongue and allowed to dissolve completely in the saliva. The dosage is usually one tablet, although for some brands it is two or three. Some cell salt remedies are available in liquid form, with the active ingredient contained in an alcohol and water solution. In this case, the dosage is one or more drops placed under the tongue with a medicine dropper (usually included in the bottle cap).

After you have taken cell salts, you should wait thirty minutes before eating or drinking anything. The idea is to let the triturated dose bypass the stomach and travel as quickly as possible to the affected cells. When you need quick relief, such as for hiccups, dissolve the tablets in a glass of warm water and drink the water in quick sips.

Sometimes it is appropriate to apply cell salts externally, although even if you do, the remedy should also be taken internally. You can apply the cell salt topically by dissolving two or three tablets (or more if using a combination of different cell salts) in a tablespoon of hot water. After the tablets have thoroughly dissolved, dip some cotton into the liquid and dab it on the affected place.

Cell salt tablets consist of the active ingredient plus a milk sugar solution. Stored in a cool, dry place, they will keep indefinitely; before using an old bottle of cell salts, check the manufacturer's expiration date to be sure the batch is still fresh. Cell salts in a bottled, alcohol-based solution may be stored in the refrigerator or kept in a medicine cabinet.

Cell Salt Dosages

Cell salts come in varying strengths called *potencies*. These potencies are designated by a number followed by the letter x—for example, 3x, 6x, 10x, 30x, etc. It is important to remember that the larger number represents a cell salt remedy that is more potent than a smaller number would be—a 30x tablet of calcium fluoride is ten times stronger than a 3x tablet. Because cell salts work in very minute dosages, the active mineral in the larger numbered "x" dose is actually smaller and therefore more potent. The common dosages for most chronic and many acute ailments are 3x and 6x. Generally speaking, most ailments will respond well to dosages no greater than 10x. Usually, higher numbered "x" dosages may be considered when consulting with a trained homeopathic practitioner.

You should take the remedy or remedies required in the doses and frequencies indicated elsewhere in this book, or follow the directions on the label of the bottle. Some cell salt remedies are sold in liquid form; in that case, follow the label directions for proper dosage.

Should you have any questions about your condition or the appropriateness of a particular remedy, always check with your healthcare professional.

Part II

Healing Yourself With Cell Salts

Overview

O ver the years, a wealth of information on the effects of Dr. Schuessler's cell salts has been documented and published throughout the world. The data provided in this section has been gathered from classic works on homeopathy, published case studies, and journal articles as well as interviews with practicing homeopaths.

Part II begins with a Simplified Remedy Guide that is designed to match up health disorders with their most appropriate cell salt remedies. By using this chart, you can quickly select the cell salt that best corresponds to a specific problem. Following this chart is an alphabetical listing of the twelve cell salts. Each listing provides an overview of the most common benefits derived from the use of each cell salt. At the end of this listing, you will find a chapter devoted to youth and beauty that offers time-tested cell salt formulas for common age- and beauty-related problems.

Simplified Remedy Guide

The following guide provides an easy-to-use listing of some of the more common disorders along with their corresponding homeopathic cell salt treatments. If you do not find the symptom or disorder you are looking for below, refer to the index found in the back of this book. This guide is not meant to substitute for the advice of a health care professional. Always consult with a qualified health care provider when a professional diagnosis is necessary.

DISORDER	HOMEOPATHIC APPROACH
First Aid	*Ferrum phos.* should be applied to the injured area in powder form. Use *kali mur.* and *ferrum phos.* for swelling. *Calc. sulph.* will help wounds that are suppurating. Silica is indicated when there is a thick yellow discharge. *Natrum sulph.* and *natrum mur.* are good for treating shock.
Acne	*Calc. phos.* is the first remedy to take if the problem is a longstanding one. *Ferrum phos., kali mur.,* and *natrum mur.* are indicated if the pustules are watery. *Kali sulph.* and silica are automatically suggested.
Aging-Related Problems	Silica, *kali mur.,* and *calc. fluor.* are of particular help to older people. *Calc. phos.* and *kali phos.* are prescribed in cases of premature senility. (*See also* Arthritis; Bones, Weakened; Bladder-Related Problems; Digestion-Related Problems; Fatigue; Memory Loss; and Vitality, Lack of.)

Airsickness	For airsickness, take *kali phos.* and *natrum mur.* before departure and during the trip.
Anemia	The phosphates of calcium (*calc. phos.*), sodium (*natrum phos.*), and iron (*ferrum phos.*) are recommended. If there is a great deal of accompanying nervousness, take *kali phos., kali sulph.,* and *mag. phos.* as well. In obstinate cases, more than one authority has suggested high doses of these cell salts. (*See also* Fatigue; and Depression.)
Appetite, Loss of	Take *natrum sulph., natrum phos.,* and *calc. phos.* before each meal.
Arthritis	This ailment calls for various remedies, depending on the specific symptoms. *Ferrum phos.* is essential for treating inflammation. *Calc. fluor.* and *calc. phos.* are often needed. *Natrum phos., natrum mur.,* and silica are especially good for chronic complaints. (*See also* Rheumatism.)
Asthma	The main remedy for asthma is *natrum sulph.,* but in this complex disorder specific conditions often call for other remedies. Silica helps when the condition is aggravated by a dusty atmosphere. Nervous asthma is helped by *kali phos.* Bronchial asthma accompanied by yellow sputum calls for *calc. phos. Kali phos.* in frequent strong doses is the remedy for labored breathing. *Kali mur.* is indicated when there are stomach or bowel upsets.
Back Pain	Silica is indicated when there is spasmodic pain. *Ferrum phos.* is needed in cases of lumbago. The two main remedies for back pain are *calc. fluor.* and *natrum mur.* The two other sodium cell salts—*natrum sulph.* and *natrum phos.*—are sometimes used, as is *kali phos.*
Bed Wetting	*Kali phos.* helps high-strung children. *Natrum phos.* is indicated when they show signs of acidity and they seem to be drinking too much before bedtime. *Ferrum phos.* is indicated if there is muscular weakness.
Behavior-Related Disorders	*See* Depression; Irritability; Melancholy; and Nervousness.
Bladder-Related Problems	If you are constantly running to the bathroom, take *mag. phos., calc. phos., natrum phos.,* and *natrum sulph.* In chronic conditions, take *kali mur.* and silica. You should

be under a doctor's supervision if this is a chronic problem. *Ferrum phos.* is indicated when inflammation is present.

Bones, Weakened

Take *calc. phos.* for fractures; *ferrum phos.* for bone diseases, hip joint disease, and so on; silica for all bone diseases; *calc. sulph.* and *calc. fluor.* for bone ulcers; and *natrum sulph.* for pains in the bones and cracking of joints. Of course, broken bones and bone disease should be treated by a doctor.

Bronchitis

When bronchitis first comes on, take *ferrum phos.* every couple of hours. In the second stage, add *kali mur.* If you have greenish expectoration, take *kali sulph.* and *natrum mur. Ferrum phos.* and *kali mur.* should be taken for all chronic conditions. (*See also* Colds; Coughs; Influenza; and Sore Throat.)

Colds

Take *ferrum phos.* It will stop a cold if it is taken at the onset of cold symptoms. *Kali mur.* and *natrum mur.* are also strongly recommended. Silica can help, as can *calc. phos.* taken at the end of a cold. (*See also* Bronchitis; Coughs; Influenza; and Sore Throat.)

Constipation

For chronic constipation, take *natrum phos.* and *natrum sulph.* If the condition is the result of over-dryness of the bowel, *natrum mur.* is indicated. If constipation is accompanied by indigestion, take *kali mur. Calc. fluor.* will help a bowel that is too relaxed. *Kali sulph.* will help in softening hard, knotty stools. Silica will help when it is hard to expel the stool. *Kali phos.* is indicated when the bowels are extremely hard to move. Needless to say, if you have bowel trouble, keep a close watch on your diet.

Coughs

Mag. phos. and silica are indicated for tickling, spasmodic coughing. For coughs that are worse in heated rooms in the evening, take *kali sulph.* Take *calc. sulph.* in alternation with *ferrum phos.* for loose, rattling coughs. Other coughs will be helped by the cell salts taken during the normal treatment of a cold. (*See also* Bronchitis; Colds; Influenza; and Sore Throat.)

Cramps

Mag. phos. and *calc. phos.* are always the main remedies for muscle cramps. Silica is also useful.

Dandruff	*See* Hair-Related Problems.
Dental Problems	*See* Gum-Related Problems and Teeth-Related Problems.
Depression	*Kali phos.* is the number one remedy for depression. You should also take *ferrum phos.* and *calc. phos.* It is best to read the chapters on these remedies, however, your own particular indications may require another remedy. Silica is also an important treatment. If you believe you suffer from depression, there are additional natural treatments available. Go to a professional health care provider to learn more about your treatment options.
Diabetes	*Natrum sulph.* and *ferrum phos.* are always required for diabetes. The first signs of diabetes call for *natrum mur., natrum phos.,* and *mag. phos. Kali mur.* is indicated for weakness, and *calc. phos.* for a dry mouth or when salt and bacon are craved. Both *calc. sulph.* and *kali sulph.* may also help. If you have diabetes, you should be under the care of a doctor.
Diarrhea	*Ferrum phos.* is always indicated for diarrhea. In cases of accompanying intermittent constipation, the sodiums (*natrum mur., natrum phos., natrum sulph.*) are good treatments. When stools are offensive smelling, take *kali phos. Mag. phos.* is indicated when there is accompanying flatulence or cramps. *Kali mur.* can help in cases of pale stools caused by rich food. (*See also* Constipation; Digestion-Related Problems; Stomach Acid-Related Problems; and Vomiting.)
Digestion-Related Problems	*Calc. phos.* is always an aid to good digestion. Silica is also extremely helpful. For flatulence take *mag. phos., calc. phos.,* and *kali mur.* Of course, almost all of the cell salts play a role in good digestion. (*See also* Appetite, Loss of; Constipation; Diarrhea; Obesity; Pain; and Stomach Acid-Related Problems.)
Discharges	Discharges are accompanied by telltale signs indicating a need for a specific cell salt. Constipation, skin sores, and asthma tend to have discharges of characteristic colors. *Natrum mur.* is indicated when the discharge is clear. *Ferrum phos.* and *calc. fluor.* are indicated when the discharge is bloody. *Kali mur.* is indicated when the discharge is grayish. *Natrum phos., kali mur.,* and *kali sulph.* are indicated when the discharge is

	yellow. *Natrum sulph.* is indicated when the discharge is green. If discharges taste sour, take *natrum phos.*
Dizziness	*Ferrum phos.* will help ease dizziness. *Kali phos.* is also recommended.
Ear-Related Problems	*Ferrum phos.* and *mag. phos.* are recommended for inflammation and pain. *Natrum mur.* and *kali phos.* are indicated in cases of dull hearing. Take *kali mur.* for swelling and earaches that seem to be located in the middle ear. For discharges take *calc. phos.* and *calc. sulph.* Children's earaches respond well to *kali sulph.* Again, at the first sign of ear swelling, call your doctor.
Eating Disorders	*See* Appetite, Loss of; Digestion-Related Problems; Gas; Obesity; and Stomach Acid-Related Problems.
Enuresis	*See* Bed Wetting.
Eye-Related Problems	After you have consulted your doctor about any eye problems of a serious nature, you may take silica along with whatever treatment is suggested. Taken with *ferrum phos.*, it helps ease inflammation and conjunctivitis. If you have pus, use *kali mur.* or *natrum phos.* if the pus is yellow. Silica and *natrum mur.* are indicated for cataracts. Other cell salt remedies for the eyes include *calc. phos.*, *calc. sulph.*, and *calc. fluor.* When nervousness is involved, the phosphates can help. *Natrum mur.* and *calc. sulph.* are indicated for double vision.
Fatigue	Nervous exhaustion and general debility are aspects of fatigue. Try *calc. phos.*, *kali phos.*, and *ferrum phos.* for fatigue. One authority also suggests silica in the 30x dose in the evenings before you go to sleep. Silica should be taken twice a week. (*See also* Depression; Insomnia; and Nervousness.)
Fingernails, Splitting	Silica is the main remedy for splitting fingernails. Read the section on beauty and silica found on page 106.
Gas	For flatulence take *mag. phos.*, *calc. phos.*, and *kali mur.* (*See also* Digestion-Related Problems.)
Gout	During inflammatory stages and at the onset take *ferrum phos.* *Natrum sulph.* is the principal remedy, but *natrum phos.* is also called for, especially when there is profuse and sour sweating. *Mag. phos.* and *kali mur.* are indicated when the pain is severe. (*See also* Pain.)

Gum-Related Problems	For sore gums, take *calc. fluor.* and *kali mur.* before meals. Silica promotes suppuration; *ferrum phos.* helps when gums are inflamed. *Calc. phos.* should help pale gums. *Natrum phos.* helps in cases of pyorrhea.
Hair-Related Problems	Silica is the most important remedy for hair problems. *Kali sulph.* is also useful. For hair loss, take *kali phos.* and silica and massage the head. When the cause of baldness is essentially genetic, nothing, not even cell salts, can change it. Otherwise, *natrum mur.* will often help. *Kali sulph.* should be taken for dandruff.
Hay Fever	Try *natrum sulph., natrum mur., ferrum phos.,* and *kali phos.* for hay fever. Take the tablets internally, but also try sniffing a watered-down lotion several times a day.
Headaches	*Natrum mur.* is the first remedy to try. You might also try *calc. sulph. Mag. phos.* and *kali phos.* can also be effective. *Natrum phos.* can help, too. Also remember to treat the causes of headaches—indigestion, acidity, nervousness, and so on. Read about headaches in the chapter on *natrum mur.*
Head Injuries	*Natrum sulph.* is the remedy for old head injuries.
Heart-Related Problems	Consult your doctor about any heart trouble symptoms. *Calc. fluor., ferrum phos.,* and silica are recommended for arteriosclerosis. Chest pains suggest *mag. phos.* or *kali phos. Ferrum phos.* and *kali mur.* are essential secondary remedies. Drop six tablets of each cell salt into a cup of warm water and sip the liquid during attacks. See a doctor immediately.
Hemorrhoids (Piles)	*Calc. fluor.* is the main remedy for hemorrhoids. *Ferrum phos.* is also called for. If the hemorrhoids are connected with constipation, treat the constipation as well. *Calc. phos.* can be alternated with *calc. fluor.* in cases of anemia. Take appropriate remedies for related nerve problems.
Hiccups	Try *mag. phos.* and *natrum mur.* in hot water for hiccups. Drink the liquid in quick sips.
Inflammation	Try *ferrum phos.* first, especially in early stages before discharges occur. *Kali mur.* is indicated for white discharges, *kali sulph.* for yellow ones, and *calc. sulph.* towards the latter part of the illness. Silica is also important for inflammation.

Influenza	*Natrum sulph., ferrum phos.,* and *kali mur.* should be taken every hour on the hour until the fever has subsided. During convalescence, use *kali. phos.* and *calc. phos. Kali mur.* is good for accompanying limb pains.
Insomnia	The three main remedies for insomnia are the phosphates of iron, potassium, and magnesium (*ferrum phos., kali phos., mag. phos.*). *Natrum phos.* can help in cases of restless sleeping. *Natrum sulph.* is also useful. (*See also* Fatigue; and Nervousness.)
Irritability	For irritability, take *kali phos.* on rising and *mag. phos.* on retiring, both in the 30x dose. These same remedies also work well in the Schuessler doses. (*See also* Memory Loss.)
Itching	For itching, try soaking a clean cloth in a hot solution of *natrum phos., mag. phos.,* and *kali phos.* Sponge the affected area. *Kali phos.* is indicated for itchy skin.
Liver-Related Problems	*Kali mur.* is important for liver problems. *Natrum sulph.* and *calc. sulph.* are indicated for biliousness. Use *kali mur.* instead of *calc. sulph.* if the tongue is white or gray. The sodium remedies (*natrum mur., natrum sulph., natrum phos.*) and *ferrum phos.* are indicated for fever and in cases of acidity. If the problem advances to jaundice, add *kali sulph.* (*See also* Pain.)
Melancholy	*Kali phos., natrum mur.,* and *kali sulph.* are the recommended remedies for melancholy.
Memory Loss	Take *kali phos.* on rising, *mag. phos.* before lunch, *natrum mur.* before dinner, and silica before retiring for loss of memory.
Menopause-Related Problems	*Ferrum phos., kali phos., calc. phos., natrum phos.,* and silica should help ease the symptoms of menopause. (*See also* Headaches; and Mood-Related Disorders.)
Menstrual Flow Problems	*Ferrum phos.* and silica are important for treating menstrual flow problems. In general, if there is an absence of menstruation, *kali phos.* is also recommended. *Mag. phos.* should relieve sharp pains or cramps. *Natrum mur.* lessens a flow that is too profuse. *Kali mur.* is indicated when there are dark clots in a flow that is too frequent or too early. *Calc. phos.* helps ease anemia in young women. (*See also* Vaginal Discharge-Related Problems.)

Mood-Related Disorders	*See* Depression; Irritability; Melancholy; and Nervousness.
Neck, Stiff	Dissolve some *ferrum phos., natrum phos.,* and *natrum mur.* in hot water, soak a bandage in the solution, and wrap the bandage around the affected spot.
Nervousness	Try *kali phos.* for nervousness. If you are a nervous person who doesn't digest food very well, try *calc. phos.*
Neuralgia	*Kali phos., ferrum phos.,* and *kali sulph.* are indicated when neuralgia is worse in the heat. *Mag. phos.* is indicated when neuralgia is worse in the cold. Silica and *calc. sulph.* can help if the problem is obstinate.
Nightmares	*Natrum mur.* should be taken morning and evening for nightmares. *Kali phos.* and *natrum phos.* should be taken before meals.
Obesity	*Natrum mur., natrum phos., calc. phos.,* and *calc. fluor.* are suggested for treating obesity.
Osteoporosis	*See* Bones, Weakened.
Pain	*Ferrum phos.* and *mag. phos.* are most commonly prescribed for pain. *Calc. fluor.* is indicated for aches and pains in the limbs due to bad circulation, and *kali mur.* for pains in the gums or gastric pains. *Kali sulph.* is good for stomach pains, *natrum phos.* for pains connected with acidity, and *natrum sulph.* for pains associated with liver problems.
Perspiration-Related Problems	Silica will reduce excessive perspiration and *kali sulph.* should help produce it when it's required.
Piles	*See* Hemorrhoids.
Rheumatism	*Ferrum phos.* and *natrum phos.* should be used to treat rheumatism accompanied by an acute fever. *Natrum phos.* and silica should be administered for chronic problems. *Ferrum phos.* and *mag. phos.* can help when the pains come on gradually. *Mag. phos.* and *kali sulph.* ease shifting pains. *Calc. fluor.* helps the joints. *Natrum sulph.* works in damp weather. (*See also* Arthritis; and Gout.)
Seasickness	For seasickness, take *kali phos.* and *natrum mur.* before departure and during the trip.

Senility	*See* Aging-Related Problems.
Sinus-Related Problems	*Ferrum phos.* is indicated for all sinus inflammations. *Calc. phos.* helps when there is a white discharge. *Natrum mur.* helps when the discharge is clear. *Kali mur.* helps when there is a fibrinous discharge, *kali sulph.* when the discharge is yellow or green, and *calc. fluor.* when the discharge is yellow and lumpy. Silica should be alternated with *calc. fluor.* and *calc. sulph.* as well. (*See also* Discharges.)
Sleep Disorders	*See* Bed Wetting; Insomnia; Nightmares; and Sleepwalking.
Sleepwalking	For sleepwalking, take *natrum mur.* and *kali phos.* before meals and silica just before retiring.
Smell, Loss of	Silica and *kali phos.* should help restore your sense of smell.
Sore Throat	*Ferrum phos.* and *Kali mur.* are the main remedies for sore throat. Take other remedies according to the color of discharges. *Calc. fluor.* will help, as will *kali phos. Calc. sulph.* should be taken when you first feel a sore throat coming on. (*See also* Colds; and Coughs.)
Stomach Acid-Related Problems	Headaches, flatulence, and biliousness are connected problems. They call for *natrum phos., natrum sulph.,* and silica. Dissolve these cell salts in hot water and drink the liquid. (*See also* Pain; and Vomiting.)
Sunburn	For sunburn, *natrum mur.* should be taken before meals in hot water. *Kali phos.* and *kali sulph.* should also be taken, before and after meals.
Teeth-Related Problems	If you are feeling feverish during a toothache, take *ferrum phos.* and *kali sulph.* Mag. phos. is good for pain. *Calc. phos.* is recommended for slow dentition in children. Silica is indicated generally for the teeth. *Calc. fluor.* helps correct enamel deficiencies. *Natrum mur.* controls excessive saliva. (*See also* Gum-Related Problems.)
Vaginal Discharge-Related Problems	See *Discharges* to determine the appropriate remedy for vaginal discharges. Silica will help when the discharge is profuse. *Kali mur.* will help generally. *Natrum mur., mag. phos.,* and *natrum sulph.* help ease irritation. (*See also* Menstrual Flow Problems.)

Varicose Veins	*Ferrum phos., calc. fluor.,* and silica are recommended remedies for varicose veins. Take the cell salts internally and also apply them externally.
Vertigo	Take *ferrum phos.* for vertigo accompanied by throbbing pain and a rush of blood to the head. Take *kali phos.* when vertigo is connected with dizziness and take *natrum sulph.* when the dizziness is accompanied by a bitter taste in the mouth. *Natrum phos.* is indicated when there are gastric problems.
Vitality, Lack of	Whenever you feel a loss of vitality, try a tonic of the five phosphate cell salts—*calc. phos., mag. phos., ferrum phos., natrum phos.,* and *kali phos.*
Voice, Loss of	*Ferrum phos.* is the main remedy for loss of voice. But *kali mur.,* taken before each meal, will help. *Kali. phos.* and *mag. phos.* will help when the cause is nervousness.
Vomiting	*Ferrum phos., natrum mur., kali mur.,* and *calc. fluor.,* dissolved in warm water and taken in sips, will help vomiting. *Natrum phos.* and *natrum sulph.* will help ease acid vomiting; *kali phos.* and *natrum phos.* will help ease vomiting with vomitus-like coffee grounds. (*See also* Stomach Acid-Related Problems.)
Warts	To get rid of warts, *kali mur., natrum sulph., natrum mur.,* and silica should be taken internally and applied externally.
Weight Problems	*See* Appetite, Loss of; and Obesity.

Calcium Fluoride
(*Calc. fluor.*)

A NATURAL PRODUCER OF
SUPPLENESS AND ELASTICITY

The cell salt calcium fluoride (*calc. fluor.*) can help treat a wide variety of health problems, from piles and varicose veins to obstinate backache, gout, and anal problems, such as itching and fissures. And that's just the beginning. There are many other problems that this cell salt remedy can help treat, including many psychological symptoms such as a groundless fear of money troubles. *Calc. fluor.* can help you if you are indecisive about little things which are not very important but cause you to worry anyway.

Calc. fluor. is a chemical union of lime and fluoric acid. This union produces a remedy with healing powers demonstrated by neither of the constituents alone. As is the case with other cell salts, *calc. fluor.* is often more helpful when it is taken along with other cell salt remedies.

Calc. fluor. is useful in treating many ailments of the bones and teeth. Many experts blame the unusual amount of dental ailments seen in Americans not only on poor diet, but also on a lack of calcium. There is, of course, calcium in milk and milk products, but there are indications that the process of pasteurization affects this calcium adversely.

Calcium fluoride is a constituent of the surfaces of bones and the enamel of teeth. It is also a prime ingredient in elastic fibers in the body, which means it will often be of importance in treating diseases of the skin and the blood vessels.

Hemorrhoids

Because calcium fluoride is a prime ingredient in your body's elastic fibers, it is useful in treating ailments such as varicose veins and hemorrhoids. Hemorrhoids often occur when blood vessels become enlarged and lose their elasticity. Calcium fluoride's role in restoring good health is its ability to maintain elasticity of the tissues and restore this elasticity where it is lacking.

Heart Trouble

People with heart trouble can find a great deal of relief with calcium fluoride. A dose every fifteen minutes or so is advisable if pain is acute. Of course, serious health problems such as this should be under a doctor's supervision.

Sensitive teeth may need calcium fluoride. Strained muscle tendons will also respond to this remedy. Both ailments can be treated with the remedy, dissolved in water and applied externally with a cotton swab, or taken internally in tablet form. *Calc. fluor.* can also be of great help in cases of vomiting (although you should use *natrum sulph.* or *natrum phos.* instead if the vomit is green or sour-smelling). If your urine has an unpleasant smell, *calc. fluor.* will help.

Calcium fluoride has even been recommended as the cell salt remedy for obesity, to be taken an hour before each meal in alternation with calcium phosphate. The idea is that these two cell salts will aid in the assimilation of starches and fat in the meals. Cutting down on these items is also helpful, of course.

Calcium fluoride is a potent remedy that can help treat many of your health problems arising from lack of elasticity in the tissues. Let's get down to the specifics of what some of these problems are, and how people have been helped by this cell salt.

Bone Health

As mentioned, calcium fluoride is often helpful in treating bone problems. A fascinating case was reported by a doctor who had a friend who had purchased a pedigreed yearling, "for a small price considering its magnificent pedigree." The doctor felt the horse was worthless—with bad ossification around the lower joints and malformed, bulging hoofs.

The horse was given *calc. phos.* as treatment for these problems, but nothing happened. Then the animal was given *calc. fluor.* in the 30x dose once a month for three months. The doctor then gave the animal no treatment for three months, after which the *calc. fluor.* was resumed for another four months. In that time, the horse recovered and became quite well. One of its forelegs was greatly improved, as were its feet. Within two years, the animal was sound and normal, and it went on to win prizes in steeplechasing. It was determined that its bone problems had been due to overfeeding, and the doctor was impressed by the amazing results of the *calc. fluor.* in remedying the situation.

Presumably, the readers of this book are not yearlings with bone problems, but they can take note of the implications of the story. Calcium fluoride can be helpful in the treatment of numerous matters involving bones, joints, and muscles. It is almost always prescribed, for example, for enlargements of the finger joints due to gout.

Backache

If you feel that your spine is being irritated or if you feel pain or fatigue in your lower back that is accompanied by a full feeling and confined bowels, take *calc. fluor.* in the 6x dose at least every half hour. It is helpful to dissolve a pill or two in a glass of water and have someone sponge the affected area with the mixture.

Robert R., a 29-year-old plasterer, was having severe backaches, sometimes in the late morning and other times all night. He was at a severe disadvantage in his work because he could not stand to reach above his head for any length of time. If he did, he felt as if his back were going to break. His doctor prescribed doses of *calc. fluor.* alternating every four hours with *natrum mur.,* and he took these remedies for two weeks. He said he began to feel better after only two or three of these doses, and the chronic condition was entirely gone after a few weeks of treatment.

Varicose Veins, Hemorrhoids, and "The Blues"

Varicose veins and hemorrhoids are two problems that *calc. fluor.* is famous for curing. You might find that these ailments go together. When they do, the afflicted patients have been described by doctors as being "calcium fluoride cases."

Take the case of a 55-year-old woman, Beverly E. She was a large woman, and the mother of five. She suffered from painful varicose veins on her legs and vulva. The veins on the lower part of her legs actually stood out like ropes. She was not a happy person. Beverly E. was just plain depressed. Damp, chilly weather did not agree with her. Her doctor had tried several remedies without success. Finally, he tried calcium fluoride in the 30x dose, followed by a variety of potencies over a period of two years. From the first doses of this remedy, she began feeling immediate relief from the pain of her varicose veins. Most important, she began to feel better psychologically. She stopped worrying about money, and damp weather no longer depressed her.

Gertrude S., a thin, weak, 42-year-old office worker had lumps in her breast and a terrible rectal fistula. Her doctor had operated twice on the rectal fistula, but it was still painful and it still discharged. At the first sign of cold weather, all of her problems seemed to worsen. Needless to say, she was very unhappy. She suffered from nervousness and dizziness, and her work simply overwhelmed her.

Her doctor realized that something had to be done. He decided to give her calcium fluoride in low doses every three to four hours, and later, to increase the potency steadily. The woman first saw an improvement in a sinus condition she had. Then she experienced lessening of the lumps in her breasts. Then the rectal fistula completely disappeared! She felt better than ever, put on some weight, and became optimistic once again.

Piles are caused by irritation of the lower intestine resulting in distention, often as a result of constipation. Rectal fistulas frequently develop when piles have gone too far. To treat piles, apply *calc. fluor.* directly with a cotton swab. Dissolve some tablets in a small amount of water and dip the applicator in the water. You should also take *calc. fluor.* internally. In serious cases, such as when the pain of varicose veins becomes so intense that the patient can no longer stand, doctors have given *calc. fluor.* tablets every two hours. This cell salt has also proven effective in treating problems of the vulva.

If you are suffering from irritated piles, it is a good idea to use calcium fluoride along with *kali sulph.* If your piles are bleeding, take *ferrum phos.* For hemorrhoidal conditions, take the *calc. fluor.* in a 6x potency before meals. *Calc. fluor.* can also be dissolved in water and applied as a compress to the anus, held all night with suitable bandage. In the case of varicose veins, use silica along with the *calc. fluor.,* morning and evening.

Diet and Hemorrhoids

If you suffer from hemorrhoids, although you can expect help from *calc. fluor.,* the most effective action would be to eliminate the basic cause of your problem: poor diet. Intelligent eating to avoid constipation has been mentioned earlier. Processed foods are the main villains in constipation. *Calc. fluor.* will help when your problem arises from your digestive organs losing their elasticity, but the reason that these organs have lost their elasticity should also be considered. *Calc. fluor.* is useful in constipation involving a chronic inability to expel feces. Sometimes constipation arises from nerves, and *calc. fluor.* is also effective in restoring high spirits.

A woman from Indiana, Mary S., had been in bed with sore, painful, bleeding piles. For three weeks, her doctor had tried various medical treatments, all to no avail. Three tablets of *calc. fluor.* every three hours cleared up her problem quickly.

In another case, a 28-year-old man, Norman R., had bleeding piles accompanied by a chronic inability to expel feces. He tried taking *calc. fluor.* and *kali mur.* in alternation every four hours, and after a few weeks he was completely cured. His doctor also prescribed an ointment of calcium fluoride and petroleum jelly, to be applied directly to the rectum every night.

Calcium fluoride has also been known to help people plagued

by nightmares. Other psychological problems that can be relieved by this powerful remedy are an inability to express yourself and the feeling that you just cannot think. If you find yourself at a loss for words and hesitate and repeat yourself in conversation, if you feel you have "cobwebs on the brain," this cell salt can do you a lot of good.

Eyes and Teeth

If your mouth is always dry and your teeth are deficient in enamel, which leads to rapid decay, *calc. fluor.* is indicated immediately. When your teeth are loose in their sockets, this is the remedy to use, and do not lose any time using it. Take *calc. fluor.* in the 6x potency before meals and *calc. phos.* after meals in the same potency. Some doctors indicate this remedy for children with delayed dentition.

Another use of *calc. fluor.* is in treating certain kinds of eye problems. Eye problems should usually be treated with a variety of cell salts for the different symptoms. Check the Simplified Remedy Guide at the beginning of this section for other cell salt remedies. *Calc. fluor.* is the main remedy if you see sparks or flickering lights before your eyes and in cases of spots on the cornea, conjunctivitis, and cataracts.

Doctors have reported that *calc. fluor.* in the 6x potency has stopped itching on the surface of the eye and has helped when the wearing of glasses all day has made the eyes water and created a sensation of air blowing on the eyes. In addition, one doctor reported that in thirteen cases of cataracts, eleven were cured with regular doses of *calc. fluor.*

Other Important Indications

Calc. fluor. is usually the remedy suggested for people who constantly vomit undigested food or who suffer from hiccups. It is also suggested in cases of asthma where the mucus coughed up contains tiny yellow lumps.

It is excellent for chapped skin, cracks in the skin, fissures in the palm of the hand, brittle fingernails, some kinds of eczema where the skin thickens and hardens (especially in damp weather), and suppurations with hard edges. Use this remedy externally together with petroleum jelly after washing the affected area well.

Calc. fluor. is often prescribed if the menstrual flow is too thick, and this cell salt seems to be of great value in many feminine problems. If after a miscarriage the uterus loses muscle tone, calcium fluoride is needed. In cases where menstruation is not only excessive but is also accompanied by bearing-down pains and flooding, this cell salt can also help.

In general, ailments requiring calcium fluoride are affected by the weather, as was previously mentioned. The sufferer tends to be sensitive to cold, drafts, dampness, and changes in the weather. Heat and warm applications also help. Frequently, you can detect that you have a need for *calc. fluor.* simply because you are sad or miserable.

Calcium fluoride is to elastic tissues what silica is to the connective tissues, and it is regarded as the complement of silica. In many cases these two remedies should be used together, or one can be used when the other fails to help the ailment.

Calcium Phosphate
(*Calc. phos.*)

THE NUTRITIONAL CELL SALT REMEDY THAT WILL MAKE YOU FEEL GOOD ALL OVER

Phosphate of lime (*calc. phos.*) is a major chemical constituent of the bones, and it is also one of the major cell salt remedies. It is given for its restorative powers following acute diseases and infections. In addition, it is specifically called for in all bone problems, as well as in many kinds of anemia, because it builds up new blood cells. It is very important in general nutrition as well.

Calc. phos., as a nutritional cell salt remedy, is one of the first cell salts to take if you are generally run-down. It is the primary remedy indicated for children who are not developing properly.

Calcium phosphate operates in an interesting manner. When symptoms indicate a need for one of the other cell salts, it is often advisable to take calcium phosphate also. This is because it tends to intensify the action of other cell salts, promoting healthy cellular activity and restoring tone to weakened organs and tissues. Calcium phosphate is a main constituent not only of the bones but also of all the cells and fluids in the body. It is interesting to note that calcium phosphate is a main ingredient in the most productive soils; the gardener who is not familiar with calcium phosphate is a poor gardener indeed.

This remedy can be very helpful for people who catch colds easily. If you are one of this unfortunate group of people, take one dose a day of *calc. phos.* and you will soon find speedy relief from this condition, even during cold weather.

The Importance of Good Nutrition

If you are taking this cell salt remedy because of digestive or nutritional problems, it is wise to combine its regular use with an intelligent approach to nutrition. After a change to a more healthful diet, you will be amazed at the improvement in your health. *Calc. phos.* can aid tremendously in your digestive processes, but no remedy can completely counteract the effects of a deleterious diet.

From many years of experience, cell salt practitioners have discovered the general eating habits of the people who probably need *calc. phos.* If you find that you have an unusual craving for salty bacon or smoked meat; if cold drinks, ice cream, and fruit seem to cause diarrhea; if eating causes stomach pains; if you have a gnawing, empty feeling in your stomach even after eating, consider yourself a likely candidate for *calc. phos.*

Taken along with *calc. fluor.*, this remedy has produced positive results for people suffering from obesity. This is because one of the problems that *calc. phos* can cure is a ravenous appetite, especially when it strikes before dinner.

If you suffer from indigestion, a dose of *calc. phos.* should be taken after every meal. It will help break up the food and promote healthy digestion. It will also help when there is an accumulation of gas.

Anemia

Quite often, the person who needs *calc. phos.* is tall, thin, listless, without ambition, and suffers from low spirits. Why does *calc. phos.* work so well in such cases? The answer is that a shortage of this mineral results in a shortage of red blood cells. A low red blood cell count, in turn, affects the bones, since red blood cells make up part of the marrow of bones. Anemia, for example, almost always calls for treatment with *calc. phos.* as well as *ferrum phos.*

April B., a 17-year old girl, suffered so much from anemia that she could do nothing more than lie around the house. She had no appetite. In addition, she exhibited two classic symptoms of *calc. phos.* deficiency. April had headaches, and her menstrual periods were irregular—sometimes she didn't menstruate for months. She had suffered like this for a long time. After taking both *calc. phos.* and *ferrum phos.* for three weeks, she was well enough to continue her studies, and the color returned to her cheeks.

April's case is not uncommon. *Calc. phos.* has helped many teenage girls because it combats female disorders. A common application of the cell salt remedies in cases of female disorders requires a couple of weeks of treatment with *calc. phos.* followed by treatment with *ferrum phos.* The two remedies should be alternated as long as the conditions persist.

Quite often those who have a calcium phosphate deficiency will have a waxy pallor to their skin. They suffer, as did April B., from headaches, often characterized by a cold feeling in the head. They may also suffer from vertigo when walking. Watching television may cause headaches in these people.

Women's Health and the "Pill"

Calcium phosphate is useful for many disorders connected with sexual organs, primarily in women. According to Schuessler: "When the suppression of the menstruation arises from anemia or from faults in the diet, then *calc. phos.* is instrumental in bringing on the period." Schuessler's description seems amply illustrated by the case of April B. Calcium phosphate can also be used in cases where girls are too young to be menstruating and where women have passed the menopause.

One homeopathic doctor has seen numerous bad side effects from the birth control pill, ranging from weight gains or weight losses to a malfunctioning thyroid. The Pill can cause changes in the breasts, he believes, and unpleasant emotional effects often result. He says when a patient has taken the Pill for many years, she often loses the ability to menstruate when she stops taking it. This doctor recommends *calc. phos.* in Schuessler doses for women who have stopped taking the Pill. (He also administers two botanical homeopathic remedies in alternation—*pulsatilla* in the 3x potency and *senecio* in the same potency.) The main role of *calc. phos.* is in restoring normal menstruation when women have been taking the Pill for a long time and then stop taking it.

Suzette W., a 31-year-old woman, had been on the Pill for four years and was plagued by irregular periods. She took several homeopathic remedies but got the best results with a single high dose of calcium phosphate. A week after this dose, her period began, and she has been regular ever since. Her doctor treated several of his women patients with similar results. Women find the suspense, as well as the discomfort, of irregular menstruation unpleasant. *Calc. phos.*, however, has been shown to be an effective remedy for this problem.

Colds

Calcium phosphate will sometimes help people suffering from colds. Take the case of Heather E., an 18-month-old child who had a short, irritating cough. She had been under the care of a pediatrician for some time, but nothing he was able to do helped. Her parents finally tried a doctor who practiced exclusively with cell salts. He quickly recognized Heather's symptoms as indicating a calcium phosphate deficiency. After three weeks of treatment, Heather's cough disappeared. More important, she showed a wonderful tendency to better health.

Teeth and Bones

One of the body's greatest needs is calcium, yet the modern diet is deficient in this mineral. Much of the digestible calcium in milk is destroyed by pasteurization. One prominent dentist who uses homeopathic remedies tries to get his patients to cut out refined sugars and starches. He suggests that they take four to six bone meal tablets each day. Two calcium cell salts—*calc. fluor.* and *calc. phos.*—are also highly recommended. He also advocates a healthy diet of whole grains, fresh fruit, and not too much beef. He says that an individual hair analysis can determine whether your need for natural enzymes, vitamins, and minerals is being met.

Calc. phos. is the primary cell salt remedy for children whose head bones are slow in forming or who seem to be slow in developing mentally as well as physically. It has also been recommended for older people who have trouble rising from a sitting position. This remedy is valuable for both old and young.

Children who need this remedy often have poor memories and bad tempers. They are often thin or even emaciated. They also tend to complain of muscle pains, especially in the left side of the body. Their teeth often appear to be very soft, and dentition is delayed. Their upper lips are frequently sore and painful, as are their tongues. They also have trouble with digestion and elimination.

Calc. phos. can also be helpful in mouth disorders such as sore throats and tonsillitis. Mark S., a five-year-old boy, had all the symptoms of a calcium phosphate deficiency. He was thin, delicate-looking, and quite tall for his age. He had problems with his hearing, and all of his symptoms were worse when he was exposed to fresh air and damp weather. His throat was so sore that he would not let a doctor examine it. After he took *calc. phos.* for three days, his soreness started disappearing. His tonsils, which had been swollen and red, started recovering. In three weeks, Mark's hearing problems were gone, and the swelling had subsided completely.

The best known use for *calc. phos.* is in treating teething problems related to poor nutrition and slow development. A seven-month-old baby, Rochelle N., had gums that were terribly swollen. She had no teeth yet and was fretful and feverish. Her doctor prescribed *calc. phos.* to be taken every two hours and also tablets of *ferrum phos.* to be given in alternation. In ten days, little Rochelle had four teeth and had also improved in every other way. The doctor suggested that she be given *calc. phos.* as a constitutional remedy throughout her growing years.

Eighteen-month-old Jim M. had only a few teeth and was thin and poorly nourished. He was given *calc. phos.* three times a day for ten days along with cod liver oil. Three months passed before the doctor saw Jim again, but in those three months the child's whole appearance had changed. His teeth were coming in, and he looked much better. Since dentition was still proceeding rather slowly, the doctor kept his patient on a strict regime of *calc. phos.*

Doctors often prescribe *calc. phos.* for pregnant women. This cell salt is especially beneficial for those who have had trouble carrying children to term in the past or who seem to exhibit the classic symptoms of calcium phosphate deficiency.

Calc. phos. is not only the chief cell salt remedy for children, it can also work miracles in dealing with the problems of the old. Many elderly people find that taking this remedy regularly keeps them feeling better. Calcium phosphate is especially indicated for rheumatism that is aggravated by night air, bad weather, and changes in the weather. When joints are bothered by cold, numbness, stiffness, or just plain aching, the best treatment is *calc. phos.* and *ferrum phos.*

Other Indications

As a nutritional aid, *calc. phos* deals with ailments that arise from malnutrition or poor diet, and it is important to remember that even if you eat correctly, or think you do, you may not be getting all of the benefits of your diet without this remedy. Headaches can be caused by a lack of calcium phosphate. When the head is terribly sensitive or is throbbing and burning, try this remedy, especially if your headaches are accompanied by symptoms of rheumatism.

Calcium phosphate is also recommended when you feel chilly, when you have a pain in the liver, and when there is a soreness aggravated by eating or motion. Sinking sensations in the abdomen, as well as problems with digestion, call for this remedy. Often, patients with a calcium phosphate deficiency have a large, flabby abdomen even when they are generally thin.

You will find that if you suffer from constipation and hemorrhoids that bleed and itch, *calc. phos.* will help if you take it along with the other salts that may be indicated. If your bladder seems to be weak and you must urinate frequently, *calc. phos.* might help. Kidney pains also indicate the need for calcium phosphate in some cases.

Back pains may yield to this remedy, as will gouty joints and extremities that act up in cold weather. Rheumatism in the ankles and stinging or shooting pains in the toes are still more indications of a need for *calc. phos.*

If your symptoms include an inability to sleep late in the

morning even though you are still sleepy when you awake, or if you suffer from overly vivid dreams or nightmares (especially in the cases of children), you are probably a subject for this remedy.

A "creeping" sensation of the skin, along with coldness and numbness of the limbs will often yield to the effects of this powerful cell salt. Generally speaking, calcium phosphate is also a recommended remedy in all cases of convalescence or debility. When broken bones, for instance, are slow to mend, calcium phosphate is a recommended remedy. A good indication that *calc. phos.* will help is when parts of your body feel as if they are asleep or if your hands and feet feel clammy.

Trembling in the calves and looseness of the bowels are signs of a need for calcium phosphate, the nutritional remedy. Sometimes it can help prevent recurrent attacks of bronchial asthma. Highly colored urine can also indicate a need for this remedy.

In general, cell salt practitioners believe that nearly all bone diseases that are not the direct result of injuries are due to a lack of calcium phosphate. They are convinced that calcium phosphate will give solidity to weak or soft bones. The healing of fractures will be aided by this remedy, as will the healing of afflictions such as curvature of the spine. Backache in the lumbar region upon rising in the morning can also be cured.

Cell salt practitioners also see a positive role for *calc. phos.* in preventing the progress of cataracts, especially when they are accompanied by right-sided headaches and eye pain. A sure sign of a need for this remedy is when the eyes feel stiff and weak. People with constant colds and catarrhs will find calcium phosphate an effective antidote to such problems, especially when the nasal discharge looks like the white of a raw egg.

In older people, *calc. phos.* will help cases of constipation, especially when it is accompanied by depression, vertigo, and headaches. When the bones around the ear hurt or ache and there is a cold feeling to the outer ear, *calc. phos.* is required.

Psychological Symptoms

Calc. phos. has also been used by doctors to help patients who are suffering from unpleasant mental states. When children are fretful or peevish, when the memory is poor, and when there seems to be an incapacity for concentrated thought, assuming other symptoms agree, this remedy can help.

One interesting case in Los Angeles concerned a 26-year-old man. Howard S. was mentally deficient, but he had several healthy brothers and sisters. He lived with his mother. He regularly suffered from nervous spells, during which he would tear his clothes. He was often fretful. His doctor prescribed both *calc. phos.* and *mag. phos.* in 3x doses, to be alternated once an hour.

After a month of taking the two cell salt remedies, Howard seemed happier and quieter. He began to follow his mother around as she did housework, quite interested in what she was doing. After two months of his cell salt regimen, his intelligence actually seemed to be developing. His interests increased, and he helped his mother with the housework. After a while, he began working with his brothers, who were carpenters, performing simple tasks such as carrying boards. Eventually, he was able to hold down a job and work every day.

All the phosphate cell salts are recommended for nerves and nerve ailments, but *calc. phos.* has had some specific successes with certain kinds of neuralgia. These are characterized by aching bones, anemia, rheumatism, and so on. You will note that the Resource List on page 143 lists firms which offer a combined product of the cell salt phosphates that are useful in such problems.

The Skin

Calc. phos. can be used with other indicated remedies in treating various skin problems, specifically facial eruptions that contain albuminous fluid, with yellow-white scabs. It is also effective in treating eczema associated with anemia. Freckles disappear when this remedy is used, or at least you will see less of them. In older people, annoying itchy skin can be helped if *calc. phos.* is taken along with *kali. phos.* Acne during puberty or in those suffering from anemia seems to respond to this remedy.

One doctor reported curing a three-year-old child who was

suffering from hand and skin eruptions. *Kali phos.*, dissolved in water and applied with a cotton swab, was tried first, but it did no good. A similar solution of *calc. phos.* produced a change in a week and cured the case in two months. The heat of the following summer produced a relapse, but the *calc. phos.* remedy cured the problem once again.

Calc. phos. is also one of the two remedies suggested for spasms and cramps (the other being *mag. phos.*). Doris R., who had been suffering for five weeks from terrible spasms in her legs that were so severe that she could not stand, was given *calc. phos.* The next day, she was back on her feet doing household chores. Doris R. never suffered another attack.

Calcium Sulphate
(*Calc. sulph.*)

A POWERFUL HEALER
AND PURIFIER OF THE BLOOD

Calcium sulphate (*calc. sulph.*), also known as plaster of Paris or gypsum, has been used for years in medicine, primarily for casts, but it can act as a healing agent as well. In minute doses, *calc. sulph.* is a healer of wounds and works together with silica in healing.

Skin Ailments

Since the skin can suffer from many kinds of external wounds, it is good to know that you can look to *calc. sulph.* as a remedy for these. This cell salt is considered a great healer and purifier of the blood. There are also other cell salts that are of particular importance in healing skin problems: *kali sulph., calc. phos., natrum mur.* and, of course, silica. *Calc. sulph.* is important because its function as an eliminator of waste materials makes it a key to preventing new infection.

Calc. sulph. has been used for years for making casts. Eggshells are made of this material, and farmers use it in soil to improve the color of grapes. But it was the cell salt practitioners who first realized its medicinal value when taken internally. Because it will hold water but tends to resist acid, some people believe that *calc. sulph.* acts as a protecting influence against fluids when it coats surfaces. It is believed to protect the stomach walls as well as the eyeballs, nasal passages, mouth, throat, bladder and any other organs that need protection against moisture.

When your skin burns and itches or is cracked or ruptured; or when you have liver spots, boils, moist or dry eczema, herpetic pustules or other eruptions—you probably need this powerful healer and purifier.

Other Kinds of Wounds

Calc. sulph. is found in most of the body's connective tissues. It is particularly important to the nerves and the bones. It is a powerful ally in helping some variations of rheumatism, for example. However, it is primarily useful in treating problems of the body's various membranes, including the skin. It will even help in other conditions, ranging from diarrhea to colds.

For gumboils, it is *the* remedy. When Marge W. of California developed a gumboil above an upper tooth after catching cold, she took *calc. sulph.* orally four times a day for two days. The result was an immediate improvement. When she took occasional doses of this cell salt over the next few days, the gumboil decreased and then entirely disappeared.

As an interesting sidelight, it is reported that a six-year-old girl, Dora C., who was also suffering from a gumboil, was given 125 tablets of *calc. sulph.* in the 3x dose. The tablets should have lasted little Dora ten days, but because they were sweet she took the entire bottle in just three days. As a result, she was not only cured of her gumboil, but also of the ulcerated tooth that was the cause of the gumboil! This healer is generally recommended when the insides of your lips are sore, if there are raw sores on your lips, and when your gums bleed during routine brushing.

If matter forms on the heads of pimples, pustules, or suppurating scabs—whenever a sore is discharging pus—the wound is at the stage where *calc. sulph.* is needed. Usually, this remedy is used in conjunction with silica since silica is the biochemical "surgeon." *Calc. sulph.* is also given for herpes eruptions and when the soles of the feet are itching.

In fact, you should not generally take *calc. sulph.* until after you have used silica. Doctors believe that silica promotes the formation of pus in wounds and *calc. sulph.* acts from that point on in healing them. It will actually stop a wound from discharging pus if it is given early enough, but when this is not possible, silica should be used before *calc. sulph.*

Infections

A good example of the use of *calc. sulph.* is found in the case of Barbara B., a 16-year-old girl who had a severe pain in her left middle ear. Knowing that an infection was the culprit, her doctor gave her some *calc. sulph.* in powdered form. After two days of dissolving the cell salt in a glass of water and then applying it to the area with a cotton swab, Barbara found that the pain was gone. The infection had actually been stopped before suppuration began.

Calc. sulph. has been prescribed by doctors when antibodies have failed to clear up cases of fever and infection. Before the development of antibiotics, both silica and *calc. sulph.* were widely used in treating wounds. A woman from Indiana, 30-year-old Helen C., had had an abscess in her right armpit for two years. So much pus was being discharged that she kept a large roll of cotton in place to absorb the discharge. No doctor had been able to help her until she visited a cell salt specialist. Since her wound was chronic, the doctor gave her *calc. sulph.* in the 6x potency. It took a few months for the wound to heal, but *calc. sulph.* finally did the job.

Not all troublesome wounds are, of course, external. Some of the worst are internal. Both sinusitis and bronchitis and their discharges will often respond to *calc. sulph.*, especially if the discharges are thick or lumpy. Naturally, you should not attempt to treat your infections with silica and *calc. sulph.* alone, without anti-infection drugs, but all of us know that infections often linger, and generally nothing a doctor does seems to help. That is the time to take, in addition to what your doctor recommends, either silica or *calc. sulph.*, as indicated by your symptoms.

When you have bronchitis, effective treatment will often call for more than *calc. sulph.* The handy remedy guide on page 31 describes which symptom calls for which remedy, but in many ailments the first thing you should take is the cell salt *ferrum phos.* The *calc. sulph.* remedy is primarily called for when the bronchitis involves unpleasant discharges, especially discharges mixed with blood. Again, however, the best idea is to use the cell salts in conjunction with advice from your doctor, whether or not he or she specializes in cell salt treatments. If you are discharging blood, see a doctor immediately.

We all know, of course, that doctors and scientists have yet to find a cure for the common cold. It is, therefore, best to study all of the cell salts and note where each is called for when you are suffering from a cold. If you have a cold in your head, for example, you may have the same sort of discharge that is produced by bronchitis. *Calc. sulph.* is indicated for this sort of discharge, and regular doses will clear up the mucous membranes.

Remember, whatever the ailment, if it produces pus, try *calc. sulph.* as the remedy. If your eyes are inflamed with discharges of thick, yellow matter, try *calc. sulph.* Many eye ailments respond to it.

Take the case of Michael C., who had been struck in the eye by a piece of wood. His sight was badly impaired by resulting conjunctivitis, and the cornea of the injured eye was dim. Michael felt a burning pain in his eye and experienced a constant flow of tears. He took *ferrum phos.* to treat the pain and the tears, but his sight did not improve. Finally, Michael was also given *calc. sulph.* in three different doses. Within a week he was able to see some light with the injured eye. The cornea was less cloudy. His doctor kept giving him *calc. sulph.,* morning and night, and in three weeks Michael's sight was back and the conjunctivitis completely cured.

Blood Purifier

Cell salt practitioners believe that *calc. sulph.* is a powerful blood purifier. It destroys worn-out red corpuscles, and is a constituent of almost all connective tissues. When a person suffers from a lack of *calc. sulph.,* diseases of the body membranes, catarrhs, and skin ailments are likely to result.

The role of *calc. sulph.* as a blood purifier is believed to be carried out primarily in the liver, where red blood cells that have finished their life cycles and are now waste must be destroyed. If you have an insufficient amount of *calc. sulph.*, your liver will become overloaded with worn-out red blood cells; cell salt theorists believe that this is the beginning of many skin eruptions. *Calc. sulph.* often eases this situation. Acne responds well to *calc. sulph.* taken with *kali mur.* Varicose ulcers are a symptom of a lack of *calc. sulph.* The topical application of *calc. sulph.*, in doses of 6x at least three times a day, can be very helpful.

Because of its role in blood purification, *calc. sulph.* is also used along with *natrum sulph.* in the treatment of kidney diseases. *Calc. sulph.* heals by building tissues. When it arrives in an area in which it is lacking, it lays the groundwork for rejuvenation by attracting other vital cell constituents.

Calc. sulph. has also proven useful, as mentioned earlier, in ear infections. It can also prevent sore throats and colds if they are caught early enough. At the first sign of these health problems, dose yourself with *calc. sulph.* in the 6x potency at least three times a day. Too much cannot hurt, but too little, or none at all, might well mean that you will be laid low by a debilitating cold.

Andrea R., two years old, had been in a hospital plagued by a croupy cough that no medication could vanquish. The cough had come on when she had been exposed to a cold wind and it subsequently had thrown her bed covers off. The choking and rattling in her chest were especially bad at night. One high potency dose of *calc. sulph.* cured her right away.

Other Uses

The use of *calc. sulph.* is almost always indicated in ailments of the pancreas, liver, and kidneys, for reasons that should now be readily apparent.

Homeopathic doctors have generally found that *calc. sulph.* (as well as *mag. phos.*) is one of the most valuable remedies for counteracting the bad side effects of coal tar drugs such as aspirin. It is believed by some homeopathic doctors that aspirin, while it may numb the pain, gradually destroys the chemistry of the bloodstream, leaving the body weakened and open to disease.

Because of its role in protecting the stomach walls, *calc. sulph.* can help stomach ulcers by coating the surface of the stomach. Women who want to have children but have been unable to become pregnant have been helped by this cell salt remedy. If your complexion is yellow or pasty, you should take *calc. sulph.* over a long period of time—at least a few months. The results will be worth waiting for. This remedy can even help some kinds of anemia.

One of the prime indications of a need for *calc. sulph.* is a burning sensation. People with burning feet are sure candidates for this blood-purifying remedy.

If you like the open air but are sensitive to drafts and catch colds easily, *calc. sulph.* may have more to offer to you than to someone without these symptoms. If you are overly sensitive to heat and cold, you probably need this remedy.

Here are some other indications that you may need this healer and purifier. If you have strained muscles from too much work and you have a sensation of heat surging through them, *calc. sulph.* may help you. Pain in the bones that is made worse by standing indicates a need for *calc. sulph.* If you are sick in bed and the warmth of the room makes you uncomfortable so that you push off the covers, try *calc. sulph.*

Do you become angry easily and then feel weak when the anger has passed? Do you worry about your heart, or your health in general, but feel better after taking a walk? Walking is one of the best things you can do to help your body, so take a walk—and try some *calc. sulph.* If you are easily confused, shy away from company, find your moods changeable, or worry excessively, you may be helped by fresh air and *calc. sulph.* If your sleep is filled with nightmares, you suffer from terrible fears and your mind becomes feeble when you need to think, if you are easily insulted and quarrelsome, or you are depressed in the morning but mirthful in the evening, you may be helped by *calc. sulph.*

Chronic headaches and occasional headaches have been cured by *calc. sulph.*, especially those that come on in the morning. The underlying similarity among these headaches is that open air seems to help them. Women who get headaches just before and during menstruation will be helped by *calc. sulph.* Double vision can also be cured by the remedy.

We have mentioned that you should use this cell salt when you feel a sore throat coming on. More particularly, if you experience redness and swelling in the throat, a sensation of tightness in the throat, excess mucus, and a pressing pain when you swallow, you probably need *calc. sulph.* There is also often a sudden, ravenous appetite or, paradoxically, no appetite at all. There may also be an aversion to coffee, meat, and milk or a desire for fruit, cold drinks, sweet or salty foods, or any liquids because of a terrible thirst.

Another use of *calc. sulph.* is to help in treating constipation and diarrhea, in certain chronic conditions. In cases of anal fistula, insufficient or difficult stool, or diarrhea in the morning or evening, *calc. sulph.* has been proven an effective treatment. The greatest homeopathic authority since Hahnemann, J.T. Kent, says that *calc. sulph.* is especially helpful for children with diarrhea when the stool is bloody and dry or whitish-yellow. A pediatrician should be consulted if such conditions persist, but you might try this remedy in conjunction with his or her suggestions.

Kent also says that this remedy is valuable in the treatment of curvature of the spine, when it is difficult for a person to sit up. He specifies its usefulness also in treating restless sleep caused by anxious and frightful dreams. In such cases the desire for sleep comes early, but the patient wakes up about midnight. After three or so in the morning, anxious thoughts keep the patient awake. If you suffer from these symptoms and experience a shaking chill that begins in the feet, then *calc. sulph.* is your remedy.

Ferrum Phosphate
(*Ferrum phos.*)

THE PRE-EMINENT
BIOCHEMICAL REMEDY

D iana P., a woman in her early thirties and the mother of two children, moved to the mountains, where she engaged in one of her favorite pastimes—gardening. She soon began to notice, however, that whenever she worked for a long time in a kneeling position and then stood up, she would feel a rush of lightheadedness. This giddiness finally became so pronounced that Diana felt she might have to stop gardening. Then, one day, when she was in town doing the marketing, she went into a health food store. While there, she told the woman who ran the store about her problem with giddiness. The woman suggested that she try biochemical *ferrum phos.*, which is actually iron phosphate, since the symptoms seemed to correspond with a need for iron in minute doses. After Diana took the *ferrum phos.*, her dizziness vanished. Now, every time it returns, she takes daily doses until she has banished it.

It is part of the character of *ferrum phos.* that it can dramatically cure cases like that of Diana P. In fact, *ferrum phos.* is known as the primary biochemical first-aid remedy because it carries oxygen throughout the body and strengthens the walls of the blood vessels, especially the arteries. Since blood that is rich in oxygen is essential to vital health and a long life, *ferrum phos.* is the first remedy to consider, especially in cases of congestion, inflammation, high temperature, or rapid pulse. This is true even if the symptoms seem to indicate another remedy.

However, it is important to understand that *ferrum phos.* is not a cure for anemia. Anemia is a complicated malady that must be attended to by a doctor. But Diana P.'s case illustrates something that is important to keep in mind as you read this chapter. You might need iron as a nutritional supplement, but in minute or homeopathic doses it can also help. In this form it works more subtly, but in the long run these minute doses lead to profound effects and are as health-giving as the best of medicines.

Iron in minute doses should be prescribed for anemia-related symptoms such as those from which Diana P. suffered. But *ferrum phos.* is good for almost everything that ails you because it is the cell salt most directly concerned with the blood, and the blood is the first place to look for health as well as sickness.

Ferrum phos.'s best uses may be those exemplified by the case of Diana P. Americans in general suffer from depression, tiredness, and dizziness. These are common complaints in every doctor's office, and usually these symptoms indicate a need for *ferrum phos.* Few doctors, unfortunately, are familiar with the use of iron in minute doses. And not all of them are aware of another cure for the symptoms mentioned above—elimination of white sugar from the diet. Depression and weakness can result from an excessive intake of white sugar. If you take *ferrum phos.* and eliminate white sugar from your diet, you may find that tiredness is no longer a problem.

Who Needs *Ferrum phos.*?

Signs that you need *ferrum phos.* (and almost everybody does in some way) are: weakness and general debility with a constant desire to lie down and rest, rheumatism and rheumatic conditions, and anemia. If you suspect that you are anemic, you should be under a doctor's supervision. Another indication that you need *ferrum phos.* is an aggravation of your symptoms when you are in the open air, as with Diana P. while she was gardening. Also, there is often a rush of blood to the brain, causing giddiness, dizziness, and sometimes even delirium.

Are you a likely candidate for *ferrum phos.* treatment? First, remember that *ferrum phos.* is recommended for nearly *all* problems because of the very important role it plays in carrying oxygen. But if physical exertion tires you easily and your vitality is low, if you have trouble concentrating and dealing with problems, if you have trouble recalling names and are easily irritated—especially with yourself, if you like to be alone, if you flush easily, then *ferrum phos.* probably is your remedy.

Menstrual-Related Problems

Jane P. had suffered for five years from nausea and vomiting after eating. She felt a terrible hammering in her forehead and temples, and her sleep was troubled by disturbing dreams. She was given *ferrum phos.* three times a day—one dose before each meal. As is so often the case with women who need *ferrum phos.,* she had also been plagued with an excessive menstrual flow and, interestingly, with toothaches. She was cured of her problems in a few days with the use of *ferrum phos.*

Ferrum phos. is often indicated for women with problems similar to those of Jane P., and it seems to be a woman's cure (which is not to say, of course, that men cannot often benefit from this wonderful cell salt). Debbie S., a 15-year-old girl who suffered from anemia, also had terrible neuralgia in her right side. As is typical of problems which call for *ferrum phos.,* her symptoms were worse in the morning. In her case, *ferrum phos.* produced some relief in the first two days and a total cure in a week.

There are many cases of girls like Debbie S. who have received relief from *ferrum phos.* Debbie was not plagued by vomiting—but many people who suffered from similar problems and were helped by this cell salt found that unpleasant vomiting was cured, too.

Vomiting

It cannot be merely coincidence that *ferrum phos.* helps pregnant women. For example, if one of your symptoms during pregnancy is vomiting foods, which leaves an acid taste, *ferrum phos.* is recommended. As mentioned earlier, Jane P. had this problem with vomiting although she was not pregnant. In another case, Judie L. was only two weeks pregnant when the symptoms that had bothered her for the last four pregnancies started showing up. She threw up constantly.

In the last four months of her previous pregnancies, she had had to stay in bed because of this problem. But this time she had a doctor who gave her *ferrum phos.* four times a day. Within a few days, the vomiting lessened, and in a month it had disappeared entirely. If Judie L. had taken *ferrum phos.* during her other pregnancies, she would have had an equally easy time with them.

Digestive Problems

Ferrum phos. can be good for digestion, especially if you have intermittent attacks of vomiting. It is sometimes useful in the first stages of peritonitis, when the abdominal area is painful to the touch. A patient in need of *ferrum phos.* is often constipated, which means that if you suffer frequently from that malady, some *ferrum phos.* would be an excellent idea. Diarrhea can also be involved, especially if it includes blood-stained mucus. Blood in the stool can indicate a serious problem. If you have blood in your stool, see a doctor immediately.

Bladder Problems

In another pregnancy-related case, a 35-year-old woman, Michelle K., could not hold her urine. She suffered mostly during the day, passing quantities of water quite involuntarily. A month after she began taking *ferrum phos.*, she was cured. Nine months later, although not pregnant, she began having the same trouble. Her visits to the restroom were far too frequent. Renewed *ferrum phos.* treatment cured her problem once and for all.

Interestingly enough, one of the provings of *ferrum phos.* is a frequent desire to urinate due to bladder inflammation. *Ferrum phos.* also helps when urine is lost during coughing.

Colds

Whenever you feel a cold coming on, you should immediately reach for *ferrum phos.* The symptoms that *ferrum phos.* has created in homeopathic provings are similar to cold symptoms: a run-down feeling, depression, a desire to be alone, and vomiting.

Some biochemists believe that a lack of *ferrum phos.* is often the cause of the common cold. When there is an iron deficiency, the blood is drawn away from the skin and outlying parts of the body so that it can concentrate in important areas such as the heart, lungs, liver, brain, and stomach. The pores of the skin are consequently closed, and there is an accumulation of non-functional matter thrown out by the mucous membranes. This accumulation is the cause of the characteristic discharges of colds, pneumonia, and pleurisy. This is why you should always think of *ferrum phos.* when you feel the scratchy throat, hot forehead, and runny nose that signal the start of a cold.

Often, people come down with colds when they are tired or discouraged. In these cases, the treatment for the cold happily coincides with the treatment for their depressed feelings. It appears that people have some control over the conditions that allow the cold virus to flourish. The viruses are real enough, of course, and that is the main reason that doctors recommend bed rest for colds.

Obviously, if despite your treatment with *ferrum phos.* and other cell salts the infection survives for more than a few days, or if your health changes radically, indicating serious complications, you should call your doctor. Generally, however, colds do not develop into pneumonia by themselves. The infections are not the same, and one does not automatically produce the other.

A former head of the Vicks Laboratories once testified in front of a Senate hearing on health that chicken soup, sympathy, and rest were still the best cold remedies. He said that most of the commercial preparations on the market actually make a cold worse if they do anything at all. This expert, unfortunately, did not know about *ferrum phos.* and the other biochemical remedies for colds, but what he said indicates something about the power of positive healing.

Simply tell yourself that you will recover soon, and you will. Although colds are a nuisance, and sometimes very unpleasant, many people frankly enjoy the attention that a cold will get them. For such people, colds may be a blessing in disguise.

When you get a cold, you might try some of the prepackaged biochemical cold remedies. Numerous manufacturers offer specialized cell salt combinations which treat the symptoms of the common cold and flu.

Ferrum phos. helps with bronchitis, too. When Louise S. of San Francisco had bouts of bronchitis and even pneumonia for several winters, she tried many remedies with no results. But then she took a biochemical solution that contained *ferrum phos.* She alternated taking *ferrum phos.* with taking *kali phos.* every hour for her exhaustion. After a thorough examination, her doctor was impressed. He said her bronchial symptoms had simply gone away.

Fevers

Ferrum phos. is said to have a great effect on fevers. Cell salt advocates believe that illness is produced by erratic molecular movements rather than by measurable deficiencies, and a fever occurs when the molecules within the body speed up too much. *Ferrum phos.* tempers the human body to make it less hard and more yielding, or more elastic.

It is usually best to use *ferrum phos.* with other cell salts. You can decide whether it might be needed for you by studying the symptoms described in this chapter. Some people believe that where *ferrum phos.* is needed so are certain other cell salt remedies, because of their close connection with it. *Kali mur.* is one of these co-workers, as is *kali phos.*

Ferrum phos. is helpful in so many cases that one is almost tempted to prescribe it generally as a preventative of health problems. Just as an example, at an important New York conference, Dr. Garth W. Boericke described *ferrum phos.* as "the children's antibiotic." It serves best, he said, where there is fever, congestion, and coughing, especially in the young.

Loss of voice

Ferrum phos. is especially recommended for loss of voice or hoarseness due to irritation of the throat. A 52-year-old minister, Tim S., was unable to address his congregation because he had lost his voice after sleeping overnight in a damp room. He took ten tablets a day of *ferrum phos.* and was cured in a short time.

Rheumatism

Ferrum phos. is also a biochemical remedy for rheumatism. One morning Mathilda J., a 42-year-old woman, awoke with an acute pain in her right upper arm and shoulder. The previous evening, Mathilda had walked through a damp meadow and had gotten her feet wet. She found that if she moved her arm gently, the pain was not too bad, but if she moved it quickly, the pain was awful. For the next several nights, Mathilda J. was doused in perspiration, and her pain became steadily worse, particularly in wet weather. Her right hand lost all strength so that she could not lift anything. At the same time, her doctor noticed that she seemed to be suffering from anemia, so he recommended that she take *ferrum phos.* Within six days, Mathilda had completely recovered, even though more wet weather was setting in.

Magnesium Phosphate (*Mag. phos.*)

AN AMAZING ANTISPASMODIC REMEDY

Magnesium phosphate (*mag. phos.*) is one of the most remarkable cell salt remedies. While it is very powerful by itself, it is also closely allied with the two other phosphate cell salts—*calc. phos.* and *kali phos.* All of the phosphates are prescribed for ailments of the nerves. It is as a result of our nerves that we feel pain, and when the nerves themselves are affected and thus cause pain, the result is doubly miserable.

A Healthy Team

Kali phos. operates on the gray nerve fibers, and *mag. phos.* operates on the white ones. But the two are closely connected, and if there is a disturbance of the molecules of the gray fibers, there will also almost inevitably be a disturbance of the white fibers as well. Many cell salt practitioners, therefore, do not give one cell salt remedy without the other. Also, as you will discover in reading the next three chapters, the ailments that the three phosphates tend to cure are related.

Although the phosphates are often used to treat similar ailments, it is important to understand the differences between them. Calcium and magnesium belong to the same group of elements, the "earth alkalis," which also include barium and strontium. The ions of magnesium and calcium are "synergistic"; that is, they produce certain reactions in combination that they cannot produce alone. In some cases, magnesium and calcium are interchangeable. But there are differences.

Calcium "tightens" cell membranes, and magnesium increases their permeability. Calcium is found mostly in the bones, and magnesium is found mostly in solution in the soft tissues. According to some experts, persons who suffer from a calcium deficiency are apt to be passive, while persons suffering from a magnesium deficiency are apt to be restless. One cell salt practitioner compared this difference to the differences between yin and yang, opposite forces in ancient Chinese philosophy. Calcium and magnesium are important elements in body structure, but sodium and potassium are important primarily in the body fluids. Calcium and magnesium reduce tissue irritability, but sodium and potassium aggravate it.

The *Mag. phos.* Personality

People who suffer from a magnesium phosphate deficiency tend to reflect this in their personalities. They are apt to suffer from constantly changing emotional ups and downs. On the other hand, people who suffer from a calcium phosphate deficiency are apt to be slow and plodding.

It is thus not surprising to learn that the primary function of *mag. phos.* is in correcting violent ailments. Spasms that affect the connective muscles, intestines, retinas, and blood vessels; dizziness; migraines; and even nausea and cold sweats can be helped by this remedy.

People who need *mag. phos.* may look somewhat like people who need *calc. phos.;* that is, thin and weak, and they often have nutritional or allergy problems. They tend to be plagued by cramps and nervousness. It has also been noted that both types tend to have dark complexions.

Magnesium and Good Health

Magnesium is actually quite plentiful in the body, considering that it is a "trace element." The amount of magnesium in the body is exceeded only by the quantities of calcium, potassium, and sodium. Magnesium is a factor in helping the blood remain alkaline, and it works with phosphorous to rebuild the nerves. It helps harden the dental enamel as calcium does. Magnesium phosphate is needed by the brain, the heart, and the muscles to relax. When a crop of potatoes or carrots is misshapen, one of the things that a farmer or gardener can do to correct the problem in the following season is to add magnesium to the soil.

It has only been during the last decade or so that the role of magnesium in the body has been appreciated by health authorities who are not cell salt practitioners. This appreciation is largely due to the work of Dr. John J. Miller, who discovered how chelated magnesium acts as a stimulus to the creation of enzymes.

New appreciation of trace elements such as magnesium has resulted from research with the atomic absorption spectrophotometer, showing that Dr. Schuessler knew what he was talking about. It has now been definitely established that a lack of magnesium will produce such symptoms as unsteady handwriting, muscle twitching, tremors, and sweating. A lack of magnesium has also been connected with such diseases as intestinal malabsorption, alcoholism, severe diarrhea, chronic liver disease, and others. Magnesium deficiency will cause confusion, personality changes, and an altered heartbeat.

The metabolism of glucose in the muscles depends on magnesium. All of these symptoms, which modern nutritional scientists are now connecting to a magnesium deficiency, were cited by Dr. Schuessler as indications of a need for *mag. phos.*

The Danger of Over-Refined Foods

The major sources of magnesium in the diet are green leaves, whole grains, nuts, and seeds. But Americans often do not get enough magnesium from their diets because all of the magnesium is in the outer layers of unprocessed foods, which are thrown away in the usual milling and refining to which our foods are subjected. In addition, biochemists believe that even if you are getting enough of the necessary cell salts in your diet, these cell salts will not necessarily get to those places in the body where a specific deficiency is causing a problem. That is why it may be necessary to take cell salt tablets when your symptoms call for them.

The symptoms that indicate that you have a magnesium deficiency are generally improved by heat and pressure. In other words, if you suffer from localized pains or neuralgia that becomes better when you apply warmth and becomes worse when you go outside, *mag. phos.* is your remedy.

Pains in the bowels, cramps in the stomach, pains in the spinal cord, convulsions, cramps from prolonged exertion, stiffness, numbness, awkwardness—these are all ailments that call for *mag. phos.* Pianists, for example, can be helped immensely by this powerful anti-spasmodic remedy, since several hours' labor each day over the keyboard can make hands stiff.

Mag. phos. can help ease nervous asthma, heart palpitations, angina pectoris, various kinds of shooting pains, constrictive spasms of the vagina, flatulence, limb jerking, and hay fever.

Neuralgia and Headaches

Certain kinds of neuralgia pains are especially likely to respond to treatment with *mag. phos.* These pains are spasmodic, almost violent, darting, and deep. They are sharp and intense. Excruciating cramps that tend to come on in the evenings and are soothed by warmth and aggravated by cold will probably be relieved by this cell salt remedy.

In some people, these pains disappear quickly when *mag. phos.* is taken. In other cases, the remedy must be taken for a longer period of time. The effects of cell salts are often subtle, but they are powerful and long-lasting. Cell salts are essentially nutritional, but they achieve a therapeutic effect. So if you take a remedy for a while with high expectations, it will have a better chance to work over time.

When magnesium salts are lacking in the body, the result may be a pain that moves from place to place and is recurrent. The pain may show up in the head, in the stomach and bowels, and even in the ovaries and limbs.

Chris E. had been suffering from pain that darted through the nerves of her head with terrible cruelty. When she consulted her physician, she had been suffering from the pain intermittently for three days. Chris E. was given two doses of *mag. phos.*, and the pain disappeared in no time at all.

Another woman, Patricia S., had experienced a boring pain that started over her right eye and in just a few moments spread over the whole right side of her face down to her jaw. *Mag. phos.* eliminated her problem in four days. It also cured her general debility and lack of appetite.

Dr. B., who was a tremendous believer in cell salts, tells a story about a patient just recovering from a fever, who developed a terrible pain over his eye. The pain was so intense that the doctor spent four days trying everything to kill the pain. Unfortunately, he did not have any *mag. phos.* The patient's family was so worried about his pain that they found another doctor, who wanted to operate. Dr. B. pleaded with the family to wait another day before making the sufferer submit to the knife. They agreed, and luckily the next day's mail brought Dr. B. a shipment of *mag. phos.* tablets, five of which were given to the patient every thirty minutes. When the pain began to recede, the tablets were cut back to five every hour. By the next day, the patient was resting comfortably. When he awoke the following morning, he no longer had any pain.

A middle-aged man from Washington took *mag. phos.* tablets every twenty minutes when he was being tormented by neuralgia. He noticed the first real diminishing of his pain in twenty minutes. He continued taking tablets every twenty minutes for several days. Six months later, the neuralgia had entirely disappeared. It never bothered him again.

Jane B., who had gone out of town to hear a concert, was suddenly stricken with such serious head pains that she had to check into a hotel and go to bed immediately. She was cured in an hour by a doctor who gave her a few *mag. phos.* pills every ten minutes.

Mag. phos. also helped Charles F., who suffered from a pain that moved from his face to his teeth in only a few hours. In another instance, a healthy-looking young woman, Barbara C., had face aches that lasted five hours when they came. After three days of taking *mag. phos.*, she reported that the pains were gone.

Doctors have had success in giving patients *mag. phos.* tablets instead of aspirin for bad pain. Toothaches have been cured with this powerful remedy. It seems to work for both young and old.

A woman of 74, Esther Y., suffered from eczema, constipation, and stomach pains. She was relieved of all three when she took *mag. phos.* to cure a neuralgia that had settled in her face and upper jaw.

Cramps

Both *calc. phos.* and *mag. phos.* are recommended for most kinds of cramps. The general recommendation is to take the *mag. phos.* in the 6x dose before meals and the *calc. phos.* in the same potency after meals. Dissolve five tablets of each cell salt in hot water and sip the water. Repeat this procedure every three hours. These remedies should help various kinds of cramps, such as those resulting from prolonged exertion, including stiffness and numbness from writer's cramp, and cramps suffered by craftsmen or laborers who must hold their tools for long periods. Cramps occurring in the bowels and the stomach, the throat and the larynx, and the corners of the mouth also respond well to this antispasmodic.

At the beginning of this chapter, it was mentioned that *calc. phos.* can be given along with magnesium phosphate. Dr. Schuessler recommended that *mag. phos.* be tried first, and if it does not work despite the fact that symptoms indicate that it should, then *calc. phos.* should be used.

Mag. phos. has also been prescribed many times with great success in cases where stomach cramps are accompanied by flatulence. It has also been effective in many stubborn cases of hiccups, especially when it is taken in hot water.

Chest Pains

Chest pains are not to be taken lightly. If you suspect that you have angina pectoris, you should not attempt to treat it at home. You should be under a doctor's care. Nonetheless, it is good to take *mag. phos.* at the first sign of chest pain. Not all pain in the chest indicates heart trouble. Some pains in the chest can be described as "false angina." Cell salts work to remove these pains, which can be frightening to the uninitiated. If you have such pains, you can treat them with *mag. phos.* tablets dropped into a glass of water. Taken frequently, they will provide prompt relief.

A 25-year-old housewife, Diane B., suddenly experienced such severe pain in her left breast that her friends feared she was dying. *Mag. phos.,* dissolved in hot water, alternated with *kali phos.* (for the weak action of her heart), worked to cure her quickly. Her pulse returned to normal, and the chest pain ceased. A doctor was on his way, and when he arrived he said that he thought she had survived only because of the *mag. phos.*

Other Indications

Mag. phos. is recommended for soothing arthritis and rheumatism. It should be taken immediately if the pains are excruciating, violent, and spasmodic. An older man, Scott N., was careworn, despondent, and exhausted from nervousness. He could not sleep because of pains in the left side of his face and chest. *Mag. phos.* was given for the spasmodic pains, and *kali phos.* was given for his lost energy. Together they cured him of his problems in about two weeks. Scott N. became a new man. He slept well, worked around the house, and no longer suffered from the spasmodic attacks.

Mag. phos. has also helped people who have lost their sense of smell because of a cold. Vomiting and watery diarrhea have been cured with this remedy taken in a little hot water. If you have spasmodic diarrhea, the remedy you should take in addition to *mag. phos.* would depend on the color of the diarrhea. Cases of spasmodic coughing have disappeared in hours thanks to *mag. phos.* Almost any problem associated with spasmodic pain, even if there are other symptoms calling for other remedies as well, points to *mag. phos.*

If your voice becomes shrill, or your windpipe closes spasmodically, *mag. phos.* will help. It may also help to use this remedy if you are diabetic or, if in your later years, you have developed some dullness in your hearing.

If you feel dull and forgetful and can't concentrate, *mag. phos.*

can help. This cell salt remedy can also relieve the pains of menstruation that precede the flow. If you had problems with menstruation and you now experience dizziness and hot flashes with menopause, you may be helped by *mag. phos.*

Spasmodic labor pains or leg cramps in the later stages of pregnancy are rapidly eased by a dose of *mag. phos.*

Applied on water-soaked cotton swabs, *mag. phos.* will help insect bites around the knees, ankles, and elbows, according to Dr. Schuessler. Insomnia that is caused by emotional turmoil can be aided by this remedy. Intense rheumatic toothaches that are soothed by heat will also improve with *mag. phos.*, as will an urge to urinate frequently.

Like all cell salt remedies, *mag. phos.* is especially good for certain types of people. This does not mean, of course, that if you are not that type you will not be helped by *mag. phos.* It does mean that if you are that type your chances of being helped are especially good. The "*mag. phos.* person" is a thin person, with dark complexion and a lean, nervous look. The nervous look is sometimes expressed by intensely staring eyes. For such people, *mag. phos.* is a constitutional remedy, which means that this cell salt will cure many of their ailments, even if it is less effective for others. People who need *mag. phos.* will often appear tired and will sit motionless in stony silence. Or they may pace to and fro. If a person has a tendency to stammer or cry or he or she complains of cold, especially up and down the spine, *mag. phos.* will help.

Finally, here are two more indications of a magnesium phosphate deficiency: a thirst for cold drinks and sugar with an aversion to coffee and a feeling of drowsiness. If from ten to eleven in the morning and four to five in the afternoon you suffer from headaches, *mag. phos.* can help you. If your brain feels as if it were swishing about and you feel a tightness in your head, consider trying *mag. phos.*

If your throat is so sore that swallowing causes pain, you have a dry cough that is so severe that it is difficult for you to speak, or you are choking or retching, *mag. phos.* can be the cure.

In general, excruciating pain and extreme exhaustion are signs that indicate to the intelligent observer that he needs *mag. phos.* It will work faster if it is dissolved in hot water, and it seems to be equally effective in all potencies. Cramps and pains are also helped by direct application of magnesium phosphate. This powerful antispasmodic holds the key to many ailments. When it is used correctly, if can effect the most miraculous of cures.

Potassium Chloride (*Kali mur.*)

THE REMEDY FOR SLUGGISH, RUN-DOWN CONDITIONS

Potassium chloride (*kali mur.*) is subtle in its action and may be overshadowed by the more dramatic cell salts such as *ferrum phos.* and *natrum mur.* Nevertheless, *kali mur.* is as important as the others. It is an important constituent of the muscles, nerve cells, and brain cells. In fact, brain cells cannot form without this cell salt. It should almost always be used with *ferrum phos.* to fight fevers. From Dr. Schuessler's time to today, cell salt practitioners have believed that *kali mur.* is the cell salt that builds the nitrogenous protein fiber, fibrin.

In many ways, *kali mur.* resembles *kali sulph.* and is indicated in many of the same problems. There is, however, one big difference: Whether the problem is constipation, diarrhea, or nasal or bronchial catarrh, the color of exudations requiring *kali mur.* tends to be white rather than yellow, as in discharges that indicate a need for *kali sulph.* Cell salt practitioners sometimes give *kali mur.* when nothing else seems to work. It is helpful in treating chronic ailments, especially where severe inflammation is involved. It should be given routinely, along with *ferrum phos.*, for colds and other catarrhal conditions. It is also prescribed for certain kinds of rheumatism, as is *kali sulph.*

A Powerful Cleanser

Kali mur. can help destroy the body's wastes when the body is fighting off a fever or an infection. It should be given when the fever has broken and the body must begin the process of convalescing and rebuilding its health. *Kali mur.* retards the secretion mechanism of the body. If you have a white vaginal discharge or dark and clotted menstrual blood, try this cell salt together with *natrum phos.* If the flow of menstrual blood is painful, alternate doses of *kali mur.* with doses of *mag. phos.*

Kali mur. also has the reputation of being able to help your body get rid of cracking noises and stuffy colds in the head and related disorders. It is specifically recommended, together with *natrum mur.* and *ferrum phos.,* for all throat problems. It will also help acne swellings and asthma. By now you will have noticed that the cell salts have overlapping effectiveness; some will treat the same ailments as others. The key to which cell salt should be used is what other conditions are present in the ailment being treated. Certain factors must be present for a certain cell salt to work.

Dennis K. had been an asthma sufferer for a long time. He coughed so hard during an attack that he had to lean over the back of his chair when the spasmodic coughing came on. He also vomited thick white phlegm. His doctor gave him *kali mur.* every twenty minutes, and later every three hours, until the cough was gone. Dennis reported that he never again experienced another acute asthmatic cough. *Kali mur.* should be used when breathing is oppressed. It should be taken every twenty minutes or so during the attack itself.

Overtaxed Liver

Kali mur. is also useful when your liver is sluggish and when piles exude dark, clotted blood. It controls blistering when it is dabbed on burns and scalds. (Also take *ferrum phos.* to relieve the pain.) As a matter of fact, you should take a dose of *kali mur.* in the 3x potency every twenty minutes for all dull, aching pain.

If fatty foods or pastries cause indigestion, *kali mur.* should be taken to help control the indigestion and gas. Of course, you should also remember that eating fatty foods and pastries can be bad for you even if they do not cause indigestion. If a pastry chef uses white sugar to make the delicious concoctions you eat (and how many pastry chefs use anything else?), you will probably develop that sluggish, run-down condition that many people take *kali mur.* to get rid of!

When you take *kali mur.* for your liver, take it in the 12x dose three times a day. This dosage is about the same amount of *kali mur.* that occurs naturally in a healthy blood cell. A tired liver can be the cause of the sluggish, run-down feeling from which so many Americans suffer. Another way this wonderful cell salt might help sufferers relieve sluggishness is by thinning the blood, so that less energy is expended as it is pumped through the arteries.

Regaining Youthful Energy

It will take more than just cell salts to bring back the energy you had when you were younger, but cell salts, especially *kali mur.,* can help. The right diet, including enough vitamins and minerals, is supremely important. So is plenty of exercise. With *kali mur.,* you should begin to develop new vitality and energy.

As mentioned earlier, *kali mur.* should be given when a fever begins to recede. This is because this remedy is a building agent. Its effectiveness lies in its ability to help a body that is recovering from disease or infection.

Rheumatism

Just as *kali sulph.* is good in cases of rheumatism, so is *kali mur.,* which seems to ease the swelling in cells concerned with excretion and absorption in cases of inflammation, rheumatic or gouty pain. One difference between the two remedies is that when motion brings on pain, *kali mur.* is indicated, while when walking makes pain disappear, *kali sulph.* is indicated. You will also have a telltale white or grayish tongue when you need *kali mur.,* rather than the yellow one that indicates you need *kali sulph.*

A classic case showing most of the symptoms indicating a need for *kali mur.* involved a 78-year-old man, Abraham Z. He had been sick for a number of years, with a poor appetite due to digestive upsets. He could not eat greasy foods and was plagued by diarrhea, constipation, stomach ache, and flatulence. His joints were always swollen. His doctor gave him *kali mur.* in the 3x potency, three tablets every two hours dissolved in hot water and taken orally. Within six weeks, all of his problems had cleared up. This story illustrates the amazing powers of this remedy in treating rheumatism and other problems.

A 12-year-old girl, Brigitte R., had pains in all her joints, especially in her wrists and elbows. A combination of *ferrum phos.* and *kali mur.* dissolved in a glass of hot water cured her problems in only a few days. The *ferrum phos.* was given during her fever, and the *kali mur.* was used during her recovery to speed it along. In the next year, when the same problem arose, the same remedies worked even faster.

In a case that Dr. Schuessler related, Hans H. had been suffering from rheumatism and fever for eight days. His joints were so swollen that he could not lie in bed comfortably, so he tried to walk all night. Hans was given *kali mur.,* and the next night he got a good night's sleep. Twelve days later, he was cured.

In another of Dr. Schuessler's cases, a 70-year-old man, Paul H., had acute rheumatism in his shoulder and elbow joints. As in the case of Hans H., every time he lay down the pains grew worse. He was cured in a relatively short time after taking the remedy of *ferrum phos.* and *kali mur.*

In still another case, a child with rheumatic fever was cured in just a few hours with *kali mur.* Rheumatic fevers are serious things, especially in children, because they seriously weaken the heart. Any child with rheumatic fever should be taken to see a doctor.

Finally, in another case, a doctor prescribed *mag. phos.* during his patient's recovery from rheumatism, because the patient began having spasmodic pains in his abdomen. Of course, if you have an acute attack of rheumatism, you should always consult your doctor in addition to using the appropriate cell salts as a supplement to the treatment.

Earaches

Earaches can be dangerous as well as annoying. If you have a persistent earache or a discharge from your ears, you should see a doctor. Because there is a great deal of mucus in the ears, *kali mur.* is one of the main treatments for earache. It should be used along with *ferrum phos.* in cases where the earache is accompanied by inflammation or fever, along with the treatment prescribed by your doctor.

Kali mur. is most useful when the inflammation has started receding and the membranes are thickening, so much so that sometimes the person's hearing can be lost. *Kali mur.* works to prevent this by eliminating the fibrin that is attempting to escape from the body through the ear's mucous membranes.

Other Uses

You can apply *kali mur.* directly to boils and carbuncles to prevent further swelling. *Kali mur.* is also used to treat anemia that is accompanied by skin eruptions. If you have backaches for which you have taken *ferrum phos.,* with no success, try *kali mur.* Tablets of *kali mur.* can be pulverized and the powder applied to first- and even second-degree burns.

Loud stomach-originating coughs and short acute coughs require *kali mur.* Always check for a white tongue, of course. If eye problems are accompanied by a white discharge, try *kali mur.*

If you have trouble digesting fatty foods, you suffer from flatulence, or your liver is sluggish, try *kali mur.* If you get gastritis from drinking hot liquids, you need *kali mur.* Also, if you have stomach aches, accompanied by constipation, try this cell salt. If your sleep is restless and you are easily disturbed, *kali mur.* will enable you once again to enjoy a refreshing night's sleep.

Potassium Phosphate
(*Kali phos.*)

SOOTHER OF JANGLED NERVES

Potassium phosphate (*kali phos.*) is the cell salt that works wonders on jangled nerves. Nowadays, it is a miracle that any of us can keep our cool. Tempers flare, and life has more problems than ever before. Luckily for us, however, Dr. Schuessler, working in the German countryside many years ago, discovered that *kali phos.* helps to calm irritable tempers, and his discoveries remain pertinent today.

Kali phos. is the cell salt that helps people when they become depressed or when they suffer from headaches due to nervousness. It has helped insomniacs enjoy a refreshing night's sleep.

Kali phos. is the most important of the three potassium remedies in the twelve-remedy cell salt group. Homeopathic doctors around the world rely on it as a tranquilizer, as do doctors who practice Dr. Schuessler's cell salt system exclusively. This remedy is prescribed to banish irritability, worry, over-excitement, over-work, and depression—even that awful extreme depression that makes even the simplest task seem a veritable Mt. Everest to be conquered.

Kali phos. has even helped people who have suffered from grief, sorrow, and despair for long periods of time—people to whom life has seemed wearing rather than joyful. These people have taken this remedy, recovered, and begun to live happy, productive lives. *Kali phos.* is often prescribed for senility, weak memory, and forgetfulness. If a busy executive or an overworked student becomes tired from too much mental exercise, *kali phos.* can provide soothing relief.

Kali phos. appears to restore direction and order to both the mind and the body. It seems to act as a stabilizing influence when vitality is flagging in the face of adversity. It can be an effective sedative if a person is suffering from restless anxiety and fears that are almost paralyzing.

Potassium operates as a "detergent" in the large intestine and alimentary canal. It is vital to the action of the heart. Some people believe that the answer to cancer lies buried somewhere in the secret of potassium's chemical action. It is known that the "secret of life" is hidden in the cells and the chemical changes there energize the cells, giving them life.

For the biochemical preparation of *kali phos.*, potassium is mixed with phosphoric acid until the solution is slightly alkaline (as opposed to acid). Phosphoric acid is vital to brain chemistry because it combines with other substances and becomes part of the gray matter of the brain.

A Remedy For Heart and Soul

Depression is just about the most awful thing that a person can endure. Often the person is not even sure why he or she is depressed, which makes it even worse. *Kali phos.* is recommended for people who have irrational fears. Such people are afraid that a hundred and one calamitous things are going to happen to them. This is not a rare problem; millions of people suffer from this mental malady, perhaps even you.

Do you sometimes lose your appetite? Do noises, even small ones, drive you crazy until you are ready to scream "I can't stand it any more"? Does one more truck with squealing brakes or rumbling by on an overpass, or another helicopter overhead, or the kids outside in the driveway drive you to distraction? Do you dread noise? If you suffer from this sort of mental state, *kali phos.* is just what the doctor ordered.

Do you wake easily? Does your memory play tricks on you? Do you suffer from a vague feeling of homesickness? These symptoms indicate a *kali phos.* deficiency. Do you suffer from melancholy, ill-humor, loss of memory, and irritability? Do you feel a need to withdraw from society? Depression can occur during a period of self-doubt, pressure, worry—when you feel you do not know what to do. But now you do know. Take *kali phos.*

Tired of life, but afraid of death, Ben R. had been treated with many medicines—but nothing worked until his doctor tried *kali phos.* For the first time in weeks, Ben R. was calmer, after only eight hours of taking the remedy. That night Ben had his first good night's sleep in a long time.

The same doctor tried the remedy on a middle-aged woman, Alice P., who although she had never thought much about religion before, suddenly became terrified by the notion that she was going to go to hell. This thought so obsessed Alice that she had to be forcibly restrained. She lamented, tore her clothes, and stared out at a world she obviously was not conscious of. But *kali phos.* worked wonders in no time.

One doctor who believes in the cell salt remedies tells the story of another doctor who did not. This physician had been overworking himself and was going through a "nervous breakdown." His condition became so bad that he was planning to give up his large practice. But his friend persuaded him to give *kali phos.* a try for thirty days. The suffering doctor said that he did not believe in cell salts, but he agreed to try this plan of action since nothing else he had tried had helped his condition at all.

In just a few days the doctor was completely cured, although he remained unconvinced of the healing power of the cell salts and refused to continue taking *kali phos.* constitutionally. Nonetheless, none of his nervous symptoms returned, and the doctor was able to see his full patient load without further trouble. Afterwards, he began to believe in the power of cell salts.

Kali phos. was reported to have cured a young schoolteacher, Ann C., who was suffering from an unfortunate love affair. She became so miserable that she had to be removed from the classroom because she banged her head against the walls. Her doctor gave her one tablet of *kali phos.*, every hour the first day and then every other hour for the next several days. She returned to her teaching completely recovered.

Insomnia

Paul N. was very successful, with a large happy family and a booming business. Then he ran into financial reverses and simply could not sleep. *Kali phos.,* administered in the 6x dose, cured Paul—not of his financial problems, but of the sleeplessness that was keeping him from solving the financial problems.

Headaches

Headaches are not easy to treat, as modern medicine and science can tell you. In the chapter about *natrum mur.,* you learned about the major remedy for headaches. But *kali phos.* is a good remedy to take, along with whatever else is indicated, if you have a "nervous headache." Nervous headaches are often related to conditions that depress or worry you, even though you may not clearly understand or realize the cause.

All of the phosphate cell salts are recommended when a headache is located over the eyes. One should take *kali phos.* in alternation with *mag. phos.,* with or without *natrum phos.*

Headaches most often helped by *kali phos.* are those brought on by, or in connection with, irritability and fatigue. If you yawn a lot, your ears hum, and you just do not feel like staying up but your symptoms disappear when things suddenly start looking interesting or when you eat, you probably need *kali phos.* Headaches resulting from too much mental exertion will be helped by this remedy, too. It is especially helpful for students who develop headaches around examination time.

A 55-year-old woman, Jewel E., had headaches so excruciating that she felt as if she would go insane. She insisted that her brain was ruptured and that it was running out of her eyes. She had been laboring under this illusion for several days when her doctor ordered her to take *kali phos.*—first one dose and then another two hours later. After having the second dose, the headaches simply disappeared.

In another case, Robin M. was suffering from a headache on the second day of her menstrual period. Immediately after she took the *kali phos.* prescribed by her doctor, her menstrual flow increased and her headache vanished.

A medical student, Robert S., was experiencing roaring and buzzing in his ears that resulted from excessive study. A doctor prescribed twelve *kali phos.* tablets, and told Robert to take one every three hours. Robert reported immediate relief, and the headaches that always came on when he exerted his brain too much were no longer a problem.

Other Indications

Generally, symptoms requiring *kali phos.* are worse in the morning and evening and persist into the night. The person suffering from these symptoms will often find that he or she feels better after getting up and slowly walking around. Cold air makes the symptoms worse; fasting may make the symptoms better. Aching pains are connected with a *kali phos.* deficiency. They seem to tear downward and can be almost paralyzing.

If you are worn to a frazzle by your job; if life has dealt you a series of blows; if you feel hopeless—try *kali phos.* as your constitutional remedy. It could change your life!

If you find that your sense of humor is becoming more and more contrary, just for the sake of contrariness, you might be on the way to becoming another Mark Twain, but you might need *kali phos.* (Twain was one of many great Americans who believed in the health benefits of these remedies.) If, in general, you find that you are indifferent to your surroundings, your finances, your family, and, finally, yourself, you probably need *kali phos.*

If your vision is blurred or you see colors before your eyes, floating black spots or halo effects, your vision could be improved by *kali phos.* If your ears are swollen, pulsating, or twitching; if you suffer from a cough with your colds; if your nervousness gets the best of you; if you develop a case of hay fever; if your nose is obstructed or swollen; if your gums are swollen, burning, and red—you need *kali phos.* Of course, if you have a serious infection, you should not attempt to treat it by yourself. See a doctor.

One important use for *kali phos.* is to eliminate certain offensive body odors. It can also eliminate bitterness in your mouth and nervous chattering of your teeth. Certain kinds of coughs are best treated with *kali phos.*, such as hacking coughs, short, spasmodic coughs, and coughs from asthma (*kali phos.* is the specific remedy for asthmatic coughs).

One of the main physiological applications of *kali phos.* is in the treatment of angina pectoris. It is taken along with *mag. phos.* Naturally, if you have chest pains you should see a doctor. But after you have seen your doctor and he or she has begun treatment, you should go to your health food store or homeopathic pharmacy and buy some *kali phos.* Everything connected with heart trouble can be treated with this cell salt—in conjunction, of course, with whatever your own physician prescribes. When the heart is full of fat or is degenerating, the lungs are inflamed, or there is pain in the chest, this wonderful soother should be taken on a regular basis.

Potassium Sulphate
(*Kali sulph.*)

A POWERFUL CARRIER
OF OXYGEN

Though its effects are often not as dramatic as those of other cell salts, potassium sulphate (*kali sulph.*) is very helpful in performing important functions. There are some indications that this cell salt can relieve baldness, although the user would have to give it plenty of time to take effect and take it along with his particular constitutional cell salt. Remember, taking your proper constitutional cell salt can be just as important in dealing with a health problem as taking the remedy called for by your particular symptoms.

Kali sulph. is the biochemical cure for dandruff, and it is very important for healthy skin. You can also use it for more serious ailments, such as rheumatism and asthma.

Ferrum phos. and *kali sulph.* work together in your body to help your blood carry oxygen to all of your cells. *Ferrum phos.* is said to regulate the "external breathing" and *kali sulph.* the "internal breathing" of cells in the exchange of gases. Both salts act in carrying oxygen, although some people believe that *kali sulph.* can carry oxygen where *ferrum phos.* cannot.

The *kali sulph.* cell salt is credited with building new skin cells, which is quite helpful in cases where the old ones have been damaged or killed due to disease. This remedy is nearly always prescribed, together with some other important cell salts, for the treatment of skin problems. (See the Simplified Remedy Guide on page 31 for examples.)

Kali sulph. and *Pulsatilla*

Kali sulph. has a strong relationship with *pulsatilla*, an important homeopathic remedy. *Pulsatilla* is a more complex compound than *kali sulph.*, however, *kali sulph.*, *kali phos.*, *calc. sulph.*, and possibly silica are the active homeopathic agents. Of these ingredients, *kali sulph.* is the dominant one.

The symptoms (such as a need for fresh air) indicating a need for *kali sulph.* or *pulsatilla* are remarkably similar. And the two remedies help similar ailments. *Kali sulph.* is to biochemical medicine what *pulsatilla* is to homeopathic medicine. Dr. Schuessler's theory is that the active ingredients in many homeopathic botanical remedies are probably the twelve cell salts.

Both *kali sulph.* and *pulsatilla*, for example, are useful in treating vertigo, when just looking up makes the patient feel as if he or she is falling. If you have a constricting headache that makes you feel as if a metal band has been put around your head, as if your head were in a vise, the doctor could prescribe either *pulsatilla* or *kali sulph.*, depending on other indications.

If you need *kali sulph.* or *pulsatilla*, standing still or lying down makes you feel worse, and you probably have eye problems—dim vision, dark colors before the eyes, and itchy, swollen eyelids. You may feel that you have lost your sense of smell, or you may suffer from a toothache. *Kali sulph.* is an important remedy for a dry, mucus-fulled sore throat in the morning and difficulties in swallowing, and *pulsatilla* helps these symptoms too.

Kali sulph. is especially effective in treating hoarseness that becomes worse in the evening. Both *kali sulph.* and *pulsatilla* are used in cases of irregular menstruation, heart palpitations, and pimples. The only difference between the two is that patients who need *kali sulph.* are obstinate, while patients who need *pulsatilla* are milder in temperament.

Hair and Skin

Older people tend to suffer from dry skin. *Kali sulph.* is a lubricating agent in the body, and it can help the skin when the necessary oils have dried up. It has been used in treating sticky and scaly dandruff, eczema, and hot, dry, harsh skin. It is always recommended for children, as a way of keeping their skin healthy during illness.

Kali sulph. is good for burning and itching hands and for crawling, stinging sensations in the skin. The remedy, which can be taken orally as a constitutional remedy or dissolved in water and applied directly with a cotton swab, will aid in removing or curing liver spots, herpes eruptions, pimples, psoriasis, and scaly eruptions arising from a moist face. There have been reports of *kali sulph.* curing ringworm.

In all skin conditions, one's emotional state is a big factor. Therefore, be sure that the remedy for your mental state is being used concurrently. If your mental state also indicates that you need *kali sulph.*, so much the better. Then you really know you are using the correct remedy.

Often, when a *kali sulph.* deficiency shows up, it does so as yellowish, slimy matter emerging out of papules on the skin. It is believed that *kali sulph.* clears up such conditions, as it carries oxygen and destroys worn-out cells. In this, it works with *ferrum phos.* Thus, in many skin inflammations, as well as in internal inflammations, *kali sulph.* is definitely the remedy.

Treat skin problems with *kali sulph.* three times a day in the 6x potency, by mouth or applied to the skin. *Kali sulph.* will help painful warts, fungus rashes, and painful, red eruptions, as well as measles-like rashes and dry skin. Eczema responds well to this remedy when the discharge is yellowish. In cases of dandruff that can be helped by *kali sulph.*, another related symptom is often a dry and scaly lower lip. Another indication of a need for *kali sulph.* is a yellowish tongue.

Mike P. had been plagued by a recurring case of small red pimples that ran together, making his face look swollen. He had suffered from this problem for five years. He had originally found some relief by using cold water, but as time went on the irritation was relieved mostly by heat. He also suffered from constipation. After trying several remedies unsuccessfully, Mike's doctor gave him *kali sulph.*, which brought about a noticeable improvement in just three days. His constipation also cleared up.

Lydia P. suffered aftereffects from a severe case of poison ivy that had lasted eight months. She had small, hard vesicles on her face, which formed thin scabs. Two doses of *kali sulph.*, dissolved in water and applied with a cotton swab morning and evening for four days, cured the case in just four weeks.

A case of baldness was also reported to be cured by this cell salt. The sufferer, Larry D., who had once had black hair all over his face and scalp, had started losing his hair by the handfuls after a case of gonorrhea. Pretty soon he had a bald spot the size of a silver dollar. He tried various treatments for several months with no effect, but a vial of *kali sulph.*, with doses taken every third day for three weeks, eliminated the bald spot. Larry's hair grew back completely as a result of this cell salt remedy.

Rheumatism

If you have pains in your joints that are eased when you walk in the open air, you may have the sort of rheumatism that can be helped by *kali sulph.* If you have pain in the lumbar region of your back during menstruation while sitting, or even while walking, *kali sulph.* is the cell salt treatment indicated. If you need *kali sulph.*, your pains will seem to "wander around," and your hands and feet will feel cold.

Rheumatism is a complex disease, of course, so you must check your symptoms carefully in the Simplified Remedy Guide. If you have headaches in a warm atmosphere and in the evening and your back, neck, and limbs ache, try *kali sulph.* Give it time to work. Some people feel it is a miracle-worker in cases of rheumatism.

Another sign that you might need *kali sulph.* for your rheumatism is experiencing restless sleeping after three or so in the morning because of soreness. Getting up and walking around will usually make things worse. This is the time to take *kali sulph.* so that you can get back to bed and have a restful night's sleep.

Carol Z., a 22-year-old woman, suffered from indigestion and general debility, including rheumatic pains. She had neuralgia in her face, which felt better when she stood at an open window and worse in stuffy, hot rooms. *Kali sulph.* relieved her condition so well that she subsequently kept a bottle around the house in case any of her old symptoms returned.

A 26-year-old lumberjack, Jerry P., was usually very healthy but caught cold while perspiring heavily after doing some hard work. He subsequently developed terrible rheumatism in his joints, which was accompanied by a high fever. The pain seemed to wander, going from his bottom to his left knee. The pain was severe, and nothing his doctor gave him seemed to help. But when he was given *kali sulph.*, the recovery was quick. His appetite returned, he could sleep comfortably, and the pains were gone within a week of starting to take this remedy.

Another young man, Robert F., lived on the banks of a lake and often got wet while fishing or shooting. Over a period of a couple of years, he started suffering from rheumatic pains after he went in the water. The pains seemed to shift from place to place. His doctor gave him *kali sulph.* to take four times a day, and within three weeks the pain had simply disappeared.

Other Indications

If a woman's menstrual period is scanty or suppressed, her abdomen feels full, and her tongue is yellow, she is suffering from a potassium sulphate deficiency. *Kali sulph.* helped Andrea H. to regain menstrual regularity, which she had lost for fifteen months after her first pregnancy.

Kali sulph. is also one of the remedies usually prescribed for asthma, especially bronchial asthma, when the lungs are filled with loose, yellowish matter that is easily coughed up. Dave M. had been suffering from an asthma attack for ten days. The attack was so severe that he could barely talk and had labored breathing. He reported a recovery only a few hours after his first dose of this remarkable cell salt. *Kali sulph.* should be used in alternation with *ferrum phos.* in cases of bronchitis with yellowish expectoration.

Kali sulph. has also been credited with helping people get back their senses of taste and smell when they have yellowish discharges. Jim W., a sailor from San Francisco, had a problem with his nostrils for fifteen months. He also caught cold easily. Three doses of *kali sulph.* once a day improved his catarrh condition in a month, and he mostly regained his senses of taste and smell.

If you develop a cough and the mucus in your throat seems to be falling back and is yellow, you should try *kali sulph.* If your diarrhea tends to be yellowish, and your stool is black, thin, and smells offensive, you need this powerful carrier of oxygen. *Kali sulph.* is sometimes indicated in gastric problems.

In cases of a yellow vaginal discharge, *kali sulph.* should be an effective treatment. However, if the discharge is not yellow or is of a very thick consistency, you should consult the Simplified Remedy Guide for the correct remedy. *Kali sulph.* also helps piles. It is a potent remedy, useful in many sorts of ailments.

Silica (*Silica*)

A REMARKABLE CELL CLEANSER

Silica is a fascinating trace element. One of the most abundant of the earth's solid components, silica comes from rocks worn down by weather into dust. This dust is absorbed by plants and becomes the supportive element, or "grit," in the plants, just as it is the supportive element in our connective tissues.

Silica is the cleanser and eliminator among Dr. Schuessler's twelve cell salts. When the skin is not perspiring enough for noxious materials to be eliminated, a dose of silica is perhaps the answer. On the other hand, someone who perspires too much and produces an offensive smell should also take a silica tablet. The person should find in a few days that he or she will never again have to worry about the problem.

Body Odor

The effect that silica has on perspiration is a fascinating one. Usually if a person needs this cell salt the bottom part of his or her body does not sweat at all. And the smell is unpleasant—especially on the feet. At the same time, this person sweats too much on the upper part of the body. Silica will help this kind of perspiration problem.

Infection

Silica is called for in more serious matters, too, such as when the body is trying to expel white pus in wounds. It is also a potent remedy for many kinds of headache, rheumatism, cataracts, certain kinds of asthma, diseased and cracked skin, and constipation, as well as the resulting fistulas and diarrhea. It is especially helpful for elderly people.

A German study of twenty-six patients showed that over a period of three months of using silica, most patients were able to avoid having surgery to remove cysts. The cysts went away totally in eighteen cases. In two cases, the silica had no effect so surgery was necessary. In six cases, the remedy helped but was not completely successful.

Silica is the recommended remedy for boils and abscesses. It is also indicated for many different psychological problems, because a lack of this essential nutrient directly affects the brain and nerve tissues.

Heat usually makes the ailments requiring silica treatment better. Cold makes them worse. If the weather has been dry and is becoming damp, expect the worst. The periods before and during thunderstorms are usually the worst for patients whose symptoms call for silica. Such patients will usually feel better when they lie down and apply heat. Pressure makes the patient feel worse. Interestingly enough, new and full moons seem to bring out the symptoms requiring silica.

Is Silica for You?

There is a general pattern of symptoms that can be found in the "silica patient." Jessica M., a 58-year-old woman, had the typical problems of a person who needs silica. She complained to her doctor of painful indigestion, acidity, sour belchings, exhaustion, depression, and spells of dizziness, which she had suffered from for years—all signs of a need for silica. Jessica told her doctor that she could not concentrate on anything and that she became easily distracted.

Jessica M.'s doctor looked not only at her current health problems, but at her whole life. He recalled that Dr. Hahnemann, the founder of homeopathic medicine, had stated that psychological symptoms such as depression indicate hidden or latent health problems. In talking with Jessica, her doctor found that she was the youngest of six sisters and had always been cheerful, tidy, studious, and reliable. She had made a bad marriage during a difficult time in her life, had come to this country as the sole support of her son, and had worked hard for many years to bring up her boy. Now, however, Jessica M. had become too ill to continue working. The doctor noted that she suffered particularly in cold weather and was often homesick for her native country.

The doctor immediately had Jessica take a high-potency dose of silica. Twenty days later she returned to him and said, "The first few days after I took this medicine I still felt bad, but then a strange thing began to happen. Although I didn't know why, slowly I began to feel more gay and cheerful, my strength began to improve, and now, for the first time, I feel more sure of myself!" She continued to take silica until her symptoms disappeared.

If you find that you have several symptoms indicating the need for silica, a cure may take a while. This is because silica is an intense remedy. It is slow but profound. The ailments it cures are often things that have been bothering the patient for a long time, such as itchy skin, acne, dandruff or splitting fingernails.

Amazing results from silica treatment were reported in the case of Jeremy M., a baby whose mother's milk seemed to be the cause of unpleasant vomiting and diarrhea. Both Jeremy and his mother were given silica and the baby recovered in a matter of days.

Silica is sometimes called the "homeopathic surgeon." Before the development of potent anti-infection drugs, doctors of the last century often relied entirely on silica in dangerous cases. We are not suggesting that your doctor abandon the antibiotic tools at his disposal, but this shows that silica is not a remedy to take lightly.

Modern homeopathic physicians note the same amazing results with silica that Dr. Schuessler reported in the nineteenth century. Soon after he described his first case, other doctors throughout Europe noted similar results with this cell salt.

Sixteen-year-old Marie R. was one of Dr. Schuessler's patients. She came to him after seeing other doctors who could do nothing for her swollen foot and were ready to amputate it. Dr. Schuessler immediately recognized the need for silica, and he told Marie to take one dose of the remedy each day. Three months later, the girl walked into his office with her foot completely healed.

Peggy H., a small, pale, nervous woman, suffered from a toothache so severe that it radiated from her jaw to the other bones of her face. Her pains were worse at night than at any other time, and she could not sleep as a result. Poor Peggy could not stand to have her teeth cared for by a dentist because of her painful jaw. When at last her doctor, having tried everything else, tried treating her with silica, her pain immediately began to subside. A few hours later, she was able to visit her dentist and have her teeth filled.

Another girl came to see Dr. Schuessler because she was often fatigued and could not think straight any more. For a week, she took silica every four hours in prescribed doses. She was noticeably better in one week and totally cured the next week.

Skin, Hair, and Nail Problems

Jack D., who spent many years working around newspapers, had a problem with his hands. They developed cracks at every joint, as well as in the palms wherever there was a crease. Jack had worked for newspapers before he joined the Army, and he went back to newspaper work after he was discharged. The problem with his hands was a perplexing one, and he had a series of tests to find out what he was allergic to. He went through six months of testing, going back to the doctor's office every week, but he never discovered the allergen. During the years he spent in the Army, the problem had disappeared. But the minute he went back to working with newspapers, the problem returned with a vengeance.

No doctor could help him. Then, one day, a friend told him about cell salts. She said that she thought that the cure for his allergy was the cell salt silica. Jack tried silica, and within a few days he noticed some improvement. After this, he changed to a new job that did not require him to be around the composing room, and every time the problem threatened to flare up again he took silica. He claims that within three days the cracks on his hands started to heal, and within a week they were completely gone.

Pat H. was a woman who never neglected her health. But she experienced problems with splitting nails and loss of hair. She tried several medicines without success and then was advised to take silica. Within three months, her hair and nails had completely recovered and looked better than ever. The results were so impressive that her hairdresser asked her what she had been doing.

Why is silica such a good remedy for the skin? It helps the epidermis eliminate wastes. Because silica hastens the suppuration of wounds and abscesses (bursting pimples and popping blisters are examples of suppuration), it has been called the "biochemical lancet." It was recognized long ago that this remedy sometimes eliminated the need for surgery.

Thus, it is not surprising that silica is so useful in many skin problems, from acne and itchy skin to dandruff and splitting fingernails and toenails. When your skin is dry and brittle and your hands are always chapped, silica is indicated. Be sure that you give this remedy a reasonable amount of time to work. Take a dose two or three times a week for several weeks. Stop the use of the remedy when you see results. Try silica any time you have unhealthy skin with inflammations tending to generate pus.

Arthritis

Silica can dissolve the urate of soda found as deposits in arthritic joints and in cases of gout. The urate of soda is flushed away through the lymphatic system (lymphatic vessels being the intermediary vessels between blood and tissues). When homeopathic silica is taken from seabeds, it is especially valuable for arthritis. During the centuries spent on the bottom of the sea, the silica becomes impregnated with valuable trace elements. In some cases, arthritis sufferers who had so much pain that they were bedridden suddenly felt better after taking silica.

Asthma

The eminent homeopathic doctor, Dr. Dorothy Shephard, says that silica is one of the great asthma treatments. When the asthmatic is suffering from humid asthma, characterized by coarse rattling, a chest full of mucus, and sweating feet, silica can be expected to help.

It has long been known that people who need silica are prone to colds involving the air passages. In chronic cases, the cough can be so persistent that it exhausts the sick person. A warm drink and silica will offer some relief. Let a silica tablet melt under your tongue and then take your drink.

Psychological Symptoms

One of the long-recognized psychological symptoms that strongly indicates the need for silica is a sense of internal sinking. If you feel a strong desire to restore your strength by eating or you have a strange sense of exhaustion and nervous problems, you must take silica.

Dr. Hahnemann first recognized just how important a remedy silica was when he realized that all people who tended to be ill-humored; who had an aversion to work and a tendency to anger quickly; or who were excessively excitable, agitated, irritated, or discouraged—needed this cell salt. A spotty memory, a general inability to think because of dizziness, vertigo, and headaches in the forehead from noon until evening, were also conditions that immediately tipped him off to the need for silica.

Headaches and Cataracts

Silica is good for a certain kind of chronic headache, complicated with nausea and vomiting, that usually begins in the morning and settles in the forehead by noon. The head often feels as if it were going to burst. Mental exertion, light, noise and cold air will make these headaches worse. So will moving the head.

Silica is also usually prescribed for cataracts, because the lens of the eye contains a relatively high concentration of silica. Naturally, if you have both headaches and cataracts you will want to read what the other remedies can do for them in the following chapters, as well as check out the Simplified Remedy Guide beginning on page 31.

Indigestion and Alcohol

If you have a lot of trouble with indigestion, silica will probably prove a helpful remedy. While indigestion responds well to a homeopathic dose of silica, many of the other salts are also very helpful in solving indigestion problems. For example, you will certainly want to read the section on Sodium Phosphate *(Natrum phos.)* on page 121. As with any condition that cell salts can help, you must study the symptoms well to know which combination of remedies or which single remedy is appropriate.

The essential function of silica in digestion is to prevent malabsorption of nutritional elements and consequent malnutrition and debility. When, for whatever reason, the connective tissue is affected, it is liable to become inflamed and damage the trophic nerves, the ones that influence nutrition.

The lack of silica in these nerves, caused by the damaged cells (which can be the result of alcohol or disease), can easily produce a condition called *chronic sepsis,* where poisons enter the bloodstream due to absorption of pathogenic bacteria from the infected area.

If you are drinking alcohol with any regularity, you are probably going to have to learn to take silica all of the time. Do not count on getting much help from aspirin. Aspirin will provide some relief, but it is harsh on your stomach walls—where damage can be done to the digestion process. Cell salts should be able to help overcome basic chemical imbalances that are caused by the physical damage done by alcohol.

Of course, one must face the fact that the damaging effects of alcohol will result in chronic indigestion even if you take silica and other cell salts. The essential theory behind biochemistry is that the organic parts of the cell are based on the inorganic salts. When the body is fixing old cells or building new ones, the presence of the cell salts is absolutely necessary. But alcohol destroys the cells so fast that—even with the proper cell salts—you cannot hope to overcome the damage it does. Sores may develop at the corners of your mouth. Sometimes you feel as if there is a hair lying on the front of your tongue. Your teeth and gums can get sore and be plagued with abscesses. Water tastes terrible, and when you drink it you may begin vomiting and feel nauseated.

To understand why alcohol is so damaging, try this experiment. If you have a cut on your finger, put a little alcohol on the spot. Feel how bad it stings. The stomach wall is affected even more by alcohol. Whole patches of it are killed by alcohol. Blood begins flowing to the area to heal it, and the cells of the surrounding stomach wall begin producing more mucus to protect themselves. The result is a raw, bloody stomach wall, and when you take aspirin to stop the pain, you are adding insult to injury.

Indigestion can mask more serious problems such as heart or gallbladder troubles or even a peptic ulcer. Plain anger and feeling upset can cause indigestion. However, in general, along with taking silica, *natrum phos.* and the other recommended cell salts, and not drinking to excess, diet is the major remedy both for constipation and indigestion—as well as avoiding the use of laxatives. Many people's problems with constipation are exacerbated by their use of laxatives, as we will learn below.

Constipation

Silica is a great help in chronic constipation problems, such as those suffered by Annabelle H. Her stool was often hard and dry and would be only partly expelled, coming partly out and then slipping back into the rectum—truly a miserable state of affairs. Annabelle started taking silica twice a day, and her constipation simply vanished. If you have been plagued with this kind of constipation, you should try taking silica in a homeopathic dosage.

The symptoms of constipation include everything from weakness and exhaustion to irritability, bloating, belching and headaches. Doctors are in a quandary as to why these symptoms are connected with constipation; they just know that they are. People who know about biochemical remedies, however, have less reason to wonder.

Another cause of constipation is that as a culture we regard the whole process of elimination as disgusting. People tend to put off "nature's call." Do that a few times and you will have regular constipation. Also, when there are not enough bathrooms for family members, people learn to "hold it in," and that habit can create habitual constipation.

Cell salt therapy, by its very nature, calls for the most natural methods of health. Take silica and the other cell salts you need to have successful fecal elimination, but remember that high-fiber food consumption and good toilet habits are also necessary.

Earlier civilizations also had constipation problems. The ancient Egyptians had concoctions to cure constipation, and Hippocrates, in early Greece, warned against using anything too strong to empty the bowels—harsh laxatives were then considered a universal cure, as bleeding was in the Middle Ages. But the problem has reached truly epidemic proportions today because of the kinds of foods we eat and the stresses of modern life.

Processed foods have little relationship to the vegetable materials from which thay came. If we would increase our intake of foods with real bulk and fiber, constipation would stop being a problem. We should simply eat more fruits and vegetables. Raw vegetables, salads, and whole grain cereals and bran help. Honey, molasses, and olive oil—or flaxseed oil—are also good. In the normal diet, silica can be found in the outer part of whole wheat grain products.

Most constipation problems are due to the modern, refined diet and a lack of exercise. You would do well to double your daily intake of fluids if you suffer from constipation. Laxatives will cause an evacuation, but they will only postpone the next evacuation. The idea is to achieve a smooth and orderly elimination of wastes at whatever is your body's natural speed.

Laxatives and Constipation

Laxatives cause more constipation than they cure. The worst laxatives are those that stimulate peristalsis—the wave-like muscle contractions that eliminate waste. The problem with stimulation of your natural action is that your bowel muscles begin to need more and more laxative to get the same effect. After a while, the muscles do not even respond naturally without laxatives. If this happens, you have become a laxative addict—with a worse constipation problem than ever.

The first step is kicking the laxative habit. Next, start taking silica. If you keep purging yourself with laxatives, the lining of the bowel becomes irritated and inflamed, and then it is really painful to visit the toilet. Because of this, you put it off. And, again, your constipation becomes worse.

Diarrhea

Silica is also a remedy for diarrhea. It became known as one of the greatest remedies for chronic diarrhea during the American Civil War. When soldiers became sick from sleeping on the damp ground and from eating all sorts of unlikely things which affected their stomachs and bowels, and they had to face long marches from the cold North into the warm South, silica was used to cure a number of their diarrhea problems.

Menstrual Discharge Problems

Most suppressed menstruation can be helped by silica. One of the indications of a lack of silica is the tendency to abort or even to become sterile. If women have vaginal discharges that are creamy in color, silica will help clear them up, especially when the flow is thick or comes in gushes.

You have probably heard stories of women eating sand during their pregnancies. Their bodies were trying to tell them something. Maybe when you were a child you ate sand at the seashore or even in your own backyard. That could have been due to a silica deficiency. According to Dr. Schuessler, a lack of "grit" can be felt both psychologically and physically. Silica is a major element on this earth, and in biochemistry silica is recognized as a very important health element indeed.

Sodium Chloride (*Natrum mur.*)

NATURE'S CURE FOR HEADACHES

One of the basic remedies for headaches is probably right on your dinner table—sodium chloride, or table salt. Of course, this does not mean that if you take a pinch of table salt, you will stop having headaches. To be effective, sodium chloride must be ingested in triturated doses—the tiny, highly potent doses that we have already described. Even then, sodium chloride, or *natrum mur.*, will not eliminate every headache. But for certain kinds of headaches, and especially for certain kinds of people, it can work wonders. It is called for in all headaches as at least one of the constituents of a homeopathic cure.

Conditions that seem to require *natrum mur.* may require, in addition, *natrum sulph.* These two cell salts work closely together in the body. *Natrum mur.* attracts needed moisture to the cells and regulates the amount of moisture, while *natrum sulph.* removes excess moisture. When the body needs *natrum sulph.* instead of *natrum mur.*, the symptoms of wateriness are pronounced.

Headaches

In 1955, in a speech before the American Institute of Homeopathy's 111th anniversary meeting, Sir John Weir—Queen Elizabeth II's physician and one of England's great all-time homeopathic practitioners—described himself as a classic *natrum mur.* case. In his student days, Sir John suffered from severe headaches, "with blindness in one eye, relieved by phenacetine and caffeine of that time, but they were no cure." The headaches would plague him for months at a time and continued to do so for several years. He later became interested in homeopathy and tried *natrum mur.* in the 200x dose, which is a higher potency than that recommended by Dr. Schuessler. "The result," said Sir John, "is no headaches in over 40 years."

Sir John believed that the most important symptoms on which to base homeopathic prescriptions are mental, experienced subjectively. He went on to describe the person for whom *natrum mur.* is a good constitutional tonic. This person becomes irritable over trifles, especially small noises such as the sound of people fussing or of a clock ticking. He or she is intense by nature, sensitive, and prefers to be alone. Music rouses feelings of great emotion. The *natrum mur.* person prefers sorrowing alone, and if a well-meaning, would-be comforter tries offering consolation, he or she is rejected with scorn. A marked symptom is a headache that feels like a thousand little hammers pounding in the head.

This description of the *natrum mur.* person did not originate with Sir John Weir. Hahnemann described these symptoms and others, such as dejection, depression, hypochondria, and tiredness of the brain. "A dull, heavy headache, especially if located in the forehead and temples, often disappears when treated with sodium chloride," he said.

Sir John described the case of a 36-year-old man, who came to him suffering from severe headaches that had been bothering him for years. After taking *natrum mur.* for three months, he was well. But he also asked if Weir "had intended to cure the bald spot which he had had for several years." Sir John concluded that being treated constitutionally for the headaches had also caused the hair to return naturally!

One should understand that headaches are only symptoms. Aspirin dims the symptom, but it does not solve the problem that is causing it. The cause of the pain is changes in blood flow. Headaches are still not understood very well, like many other ills of modern living, but *natrum mur.* appears to be a good remedy for such modern maladies. These ills are often experienced as headaches. Even antibiotics can cause headaches. Stress, fatigue, loud noise, depression, and foods that disagree, such as alcohol, chocolate and cheese, or even an argument with one's spouse, can bring on headaches.

Sometimes the best way to handle a headache is to lie down or eat something (often hunger is expressed by the body as a dull headache). However, hypertension and brain tumors can also cause headaches. Some people think that viruses are a cause of headaches. Cold also causes headaches (though heat generally does not).

L. R. Twentymen, then the editor of the prestigious *British Homeopathic Journal*, suggested to a homeopathic conference held in Vienna in 1973 that *natrum mur.* symptoms are "the mirror of our times." He stated that, "Twenty percent of the population suffers from migraines, and this type of headache is common in the *natrum mur.* personality."

Natrum mur. is indicated again and again as the remedy for headaches. A 50-year-old widow, Madeline A., told her doctor she had been suffering from headaches for twenty-two years. She craved solitude, having been disappointed in love. Her continuing headaches included a bursting pain in her forehead. Her doctor, convinced by these and other symptoms that her need was for *natrum mur.,* issued her two potent constitutional doses—the first was 1x and the second, taken three months later, was 10x. This treatment caused her headaches to disappear.

Double Vision

Marianne C. was a teacher who complained of double vision. At times, she said, she could see only half of an object in front of her. The examining doctor found that Marianne got headaches that were worse in the morning than later in the day, became worse whenever she tried any mental exertion, and were relieved somewhat by sitting or lying down. Her doctor prescribed five tablets of *natrum mur.* in the Schuessler dose every hour on the hour. Not long afterwards, Marianne C. returned to her class, completely cured of her headaches and double vision.

Eczema

A New York doctor reported a case in which he treated a bad case of eczema with *natrum mur.* Although the patient, Israel B., appeared to require a particular homeopathic remedy as his constitutional, the remedy was not helping. So the doctor started taking a personal history of his patient and found that prior to the skin condition, Israel's sister had been committed to a psychiatric hospital. Israel began weeping profusely at the mention of this fact. One of the well-known signs of a need for *natrum mur.* is excessive weeping. This led the doctor to try *natrum mur.* He says that Israel's condition cleared up in no time at all.

The Power of *Natrum mur.*

Natrum mur. is often recommended as a treatment for more serious diseases. A famous English doctor tells how his brother, also a doctor, "had remarkable successes in treating multiple sclerosis" with *natrum mur.*

Charles E. Wheeler, a past president of the British Homeopathic Society, calls *natrum mur.* "one of the most profound remedies for chronic diseases." It has been a traditional remedy for certain complaints of infants and also in cases of malaria. It cures certain kinds of anemia, "where red corpuscles and hemoglobin are deficient without profound blood changes."

Although sodium chloride is common to most living things, it is present in a much higher concentration in bodily fluids than in things such as bones and muscles. Sodium chloride's great quality is its creation of osmotic pressure. Osmosis is important, since without it water would lose its life-giving qualities in the body. It is the key to many delicate and important chemical processes in the body. Without osmosis, body cells could not be given the nutrients and chemicals they require, because cells stay in one place in the body. They know exactly the kind of nutrition they need and will reject imitations, but they cannot go hunt for it. The blood must bring the necessary nutrients, which then are transmitted to the cells by osmosis—a process controlled by sodium chloride.

The paradoxical powers of sodium chloride are demonstrated by the fact that, in homeopathic doses, it is regarded as a good antidote to hay fever, yet this same method of treating hay fever also calls for elimination of sodium chloride in the form of table salt from the diet.

Sodium, the element, has an important synergistic relationship with potassium. Some authorities believe that an overabundance of sodium in the form of table salt can antagonize its partnership with potassium, upsetting the body's balance and even causing such troubles as cancer and high blood pressure. Therefore, it is best to limit table salt intake to a reasonable amount, since it can build up in the body over a long period of time and cause various health problems.

The primary indication of a sodium chloride deficiency is either an exceptional dryness anywhere in the body or, conversely, an overabundance of water. If you need *natrum mur.*, you will probably appear bloated, feel languid and drowsy and suffer from chilly extremities. You will most likely have a pronounced craving for salt—because even though you may be eating many more times the required amount with your meals, it cannot be absorbed by the body unless it is taken in minute doses.

Heart Disease

A famous British homeopath mentions a case confirming the fact that *natrum mur.* is often a recommended constitutional remedy in heart cases. She had a 75-year-old patient, Beatrice R., who was recovering from a heart attack and was not given terribly long to live. Beatrice was not very happy with the other homeopathic remedies she was being treated with. After she observed the patient for some time, a picture began to form in the doctor's mind, and she realized that her patient had virtually all of the classic *natrum mur.* symptoms. She was estranged from her family, but rarely talked about it, hated sympathy, felt the heat too much, was tired and exhausted in the mornings and had a liking for salty foods and sweets. Her skin was sallow and yellow. Her doctor put her on *natrum mur.* in the Schuessler 6x dose, to be taken morning and night.

"The progress was almost startling after this," the doctor reported. Beatrice became energetic, started up a daily round of social engagements and generally showed more life. Her heart became stronger, and three years later there still was not a murmur from that vital organ. Beatrice R. felt better than ever; *natrum mur.* was obviously her constitutional remedy.

The *Natrum mur.* Personality

People who can be expected to respond well to *natrum mur.* cell salts can often be recognized by their free, watery discharges, which flow far too easily from the mucous membranes. *Natrum mur.*, however, is also indicated in cases where the vagina is excessively dry. *Natrum mur.* subjects also tend to be sensitive to light and heat, and they have poor circulation. They are often chilly, and their conditions appear to be aggravated by the seashore. They are often melancholy. Fear of thunder is a symptom. Sir John Weir said that during the air raids in London during World War II, a need for *natrum mur.* was indicated in cases of shock.

Natrum mur. people often suffer from constipation, hard, dry stools which tend to cause anal fissures, and diarrhea, sometimes alternating with constipation.

It is interesting to note that headaches and abnormal fatigue are symptoms caused by excess sodium chloride in the diet in the form of table salt, whereas these same problems often react favorably to sodium chloride in triturated doses. This seeming paradox is nothing new to homeopathy. A homeopathic remedy is proven by observing the symptoms of illness it produces in well people. From these observations, homeopaths can expect the same mineral in homeopathic doses to cure these conditions.

Dr. Schuessler believed that a considerable amount of sodium chloride powder, dissolved in water and applied externally with cotton, was an effective treatment for insect bites. Moisten the bite with a small amount of water and rub a little sodium chloride on the spot. Dr. Schuessler said that the pain would stop almost instantly.

Dry psoriasis will usually clear up in two or three days with *natrum mur.* in the Schuessler-recommended 6x dose. Constipation is sometimes related to this condition and calls for the 3x dose. *Natrum mur.* in the 6x dosage has also been suggested for the treatment of rheumatism (three pills, three times a day), as well as for varicose veins.

Sodium Phosphate (*Natrum phos.*)

THE BIOCHEMICAL ANTACID

Sodium phosphate (*natrum phos.*) has often been called the "biochemical antacid." It plays this role not only in digestion but also in the body's fluids, including the blood. But it is a major remedy for indigestion. If this is your problem, you should also read the Silica section on page 103. Check the Simplified Remedy Guide as well.

Americans spend over a quarter of a billion dollars a year on medications that promise relief from indigestion. Yet the best advice for those who suffer from indigestion is to change their diet and try the various biochemical remedies, which cannot hurt and will most likely help. Many antacids that people take for stomach upset contain bicarbonate of soda, which can cause the formation of kidney stones and recurrent urinary tract infections. The high sodium count of "bicarb" also makes it bad for people with incipient heart trouble or kidney problems.

The next time you are stricken with indigestion, instead of using one of the commercial preparations, eat and drink nothing until the pain is gone. Then try adding clear liquids—water, herbal tea, or broth. Next, add bland foods such as toast, rice, mashed potatoes, and the like. Music and meditation can also help, because anxiety produces excess stomach acid and the excess stomach acid produces indigestion.

Chronic indigestion may mask more serious ailments. If treating indigestion with biochemical preparations and changing your diet do not help, your "indigestion" may actually be gallbladder or heart problems, or even a peptic ulcer, masquerading as common indigestion. So, be methodical. Keep a record of your diet, recording the effect various foods have on your indigestion. Also, be sure not to overeat to the point where you feel stuffed.

It is now known that the state of one's nerves can have a profound effect on digestion. The digestive function is practically the first thing affected by an agitated mental condition. The pioneer homeopathic doctor James Tyler Kent always prescribed *natrum phos.* for patients who were "in a fret from mental exertion" as well as those suffering from "sexual excesses and vices." Kent found *natrum phos.* most helpful in cases where the symptoms resulted from fasting, as well as in cases in which symptoms were relieved by eating, such as headache. Other symptoms that he treated with this remedy included those made worse by cold and the open air and by physical exertion. If you find butter, cold drinks, fats, fruit, milk, sour foods, or vinegar troubling to your digestion, take Dr. Kent's advice and try *natrum phos.*

Indigestion is a very complex problem, intimately connected with your whole nervous system. If you find yourself becoming angry at trifles, easily vexed, anxious at night, not feeling very sociable, or suffering from mental fuzziness, all of these problems could be signs that indicate a need for *natrum phos.* The symptoms helped by *natrum phos.* in cases of indigestion often indicate other health problems.

Why Good Digestion Is Necessary

Physically, digestion (or a lack of it) is central and vital to your health. If you are not digesting your food properly, you cannot eliminate properly. Problems such as constipation and diarrhea have an immediate effect on how you feel. *Natrum phos.* can help you if you find yourself developing an aversion to food you would otherwise like. If you feel "heat" in your stomach, nausea in the morning, and pain in your stomach after eating, *natrum phos.* is your remedy. It is also indicated if you suffer from alternate bouts of constipation and diarrhea.

Even your dreams can be tied to indigestion. If, after raiding the refrigerator for a midnight snack, you dream a lot and the dreams are vivid or make you feel anxious, *natrum phos.* will help you sleep more comfortably.

A 50-year-old woman, Beulah P., had been having severe attacks of gastric pain for two years. She vomited frequently. Beulah was given Schuessler dosages of *natrum phos.*, and in two days she could feel the difference. Within a few weeks she was cured.

Milano K., a feverish lad, suffered from a sour stomach. His breath was sour, and his vomit resembled curdled milk. In addition, young Milano was cross, fretful and restless, as the result of an infection from which he had otherwise recovered. A dose of *natrum phos.* cured him almost immediately.

A doctor reported amazing success with a patient, Sidney G., who had been suffering from a troublesome burning sensation which began an hour or two after each meal and continued for a long time. He suffered no extreme thirst, and his bowels were regular, but the burning pain was so terrible that Sidney could not sleep. *Natrum phos.* cured him almost instantly.

Bill C. was also quickly cured of chronic dyspepsia. His doctor prescribed *natrum phos.* after observing that Bill's soft palate was covered with a thick, yellow, creamy coating. In a very short time, a dose of *natrum phos.* cleared up both the yellow coating and the dyspepsia.

A little boy, Jon N., ate too much candy one day and followed it up with several bananas. Soon he suffered an attack of sour vomiting so severe that he went into convulsions. *Natrum phos.* brought a speedy cure even to this problem.

Of course, you should take *natrum phos.*, or any other cell salt remedy, only as a part of a conscious attempt to follow a more healthy lifestyle. If the cells of your body are depleted of vital cell salts, it might take more than the ingestion of the indicated remedy to cure you. The whole theory behind the use of cell salts is that your body can cure itself. The cell salts are merely catalysts.

Sometimes, however, a cure may require a change of surroundings, a happy occupation, good food, vitamins and exercise, regular sleep, and better, effortless evacuation of the bowels and bladder. All of these are things to concentrate on in the event of illness. After these have been attended to, one can begin the administration of cell salts.

A Helpful Combination

In some cases of rheumatism, *natrum phos.* is called for in conjunction with *ferrum phos.* Phosphate never occurs in a free state; it is always in combination with other substances. It is found in urine and can be extracted from the bones. It was discovered in Germany in 1673, and its properties of healing have been discovered by many since then. You will find that the phosphates are included in some of the most important remedies in cell salt treatment. They are used as a standard cell salt nerve tonic, among many other things.

Natrum phos. is recommended first in cases of indigestion. But once the condition has been left unattended too long, or has been made worse by the use of patent antacids or other medicines, the general rule of thumb is to combine *natrum phos.* with *natrum sulph.* These two cell salts work remarkably together. If you have headaches in addition to indigestion and they are located in the forehead, or if your skull feels "too full," think of *natrum sulph.* If you have pain in your stomach or your stomach seems full of frothy, sour fluids, once again, *natrum phos.* will do the trick. Be sure you alternate these two cell salts with doses of *ferrum phos.* as well.

Back Pain and Rheumatism

Natrum phos. is also useful for some back pains and in all acute or chronic cases of inflammatory rheumatism. Alternate *natrum phos.* with the other cell salts called for by the condition. Rheumatic pains in the joints, a weak feeling in the legs, cracking and creaking in the joints—these symptoms all call for *natrum phos.*

The primary indication that you have a rheumatic condition that can be helped by this remedy is a yellow-coated tongue and other acid symptoms involving the mouth and sweat glands. Dr. Schuessler himself was the first to note the rapid effects of *natrum phos.* on such rheumatic symptoms. If your symptoms seem worse during menstruation, you may need *natrum phos.* The point is that the primary role of *natrum phos.* is the decomposition of lactic acid and the emulsification of fatty acids. It is found in the blood, muscles, nerves and brain cells—and many illnesses involving these organs require it.

In many diseases, the common factor is acidity of the blood. Cell salts, as you know, operate in the individual cells, and *natrum phos.* helps reduce the blood's acidity. *Natrum phos.* is routinely used for such ailments as gout, stomach ulceration, and worms. It helps emulsify decomposed lactic acid, which causes pain in rheumatic conditions. However, in most cases of toxic and acid rheumatism, *natrum phos.* is recommended along with other cell salts such as silica and *kali sulph.* For rheumatism, one expert recommends using the appropriate cell salts in alternation, three times a day.

Eye Problems

Natrum phos. has long been used for conjunctivitis, an inflammation of the eyelid, and is one of the time-honored remedies for this condition. Schuessler first noted its effect in a little girl who had suffered from conjunctivitis for several years. She had creamy secretions from her eyelids, so Schuessler administered a dose of this remedy three times daily. A week later, her eyes were bright and clear. The reason for this, it is now believed, is that the eyes are particularly sensitive to acid conditions. *Natrum phos.* is called for in many cases where there is a creamy secretion—for example, a creamy vaginal discharge.

Kicking Addictions

A physician, Dr. X., had a terrible morphine addiction. He was cured with biochemical doses of *natrum phos.* For two months, another doctor treated him by administering the *natrum phos.* under the skin as an injection. These shots were gradually increased as the morphine was decreased. In two months, the doctor permanently lost his daily habit.

Vertigo

Vertigo—a feeling of dizziness—is a definite indication of a need for *natrum phos.*, especially when it is accompanied by acid-producing gastric problems. Digby D. was a vertigo sufferer who had been plagued with the problem for a number of weeks. The condition was so bad that he could not stand up. He became ill and was doing a lot of vomiting. He was cured with *natrum phos.* in a week's time.

Other uses

Other conditions where *natrum phos.* has been helpful include restless sleeping, an itching anus, eczema, hives and rose rash.

Sodium Sulphate
(*Natrum sulph.*)

A MIRACULOUS REMEDY
FOR ASTHMA

Sodium sulphate (*natrum sulph.*), which is produced by the action of sulphuric acid on common table salt, occurs naturally in large quantities in many salt lakes. When it is manufactured, its common name is Glauber's salt; but for use as a cell salt remedy, *natrum sulph.* is always obtained directly from natural sources.

Sodium chloride attracts water to the body tissues, and *natrum sulph.* regulates the carrying of water *away from* the body tissues. Of course, this process has many health benefits, making *natrum sulph.* a remedy for many ailments—including such diverse ones as asthma, diabetes, influenza and old head injuries—just because of its powerful influence on the waste-removing process of the body's cells.

Asthma

Natrum sulph. is, in fact, the main cell salt remedy for asthma. Ailments that are aggravated by dampness, fog, and wet weather are "provings" of this cell salt; asthma is certainly made worse by dampness, fog, and wet weather.

A hard, asthmatic cough, with thick expectoration and a constant desire to take long, deep breaths, is a strong sign that you need *natrum sulph.* In addition, hay fever that comes on during a damp, chilly day or during a hot, humid day is a further indication that *natrum sulph.* can help you.

Natrum sulph., taken in high doses, was valuable in the case of Frederick S., a 10-year-old, shy, intelligent, and restless lad, who had so many attacks of asthma that his family never got a good night's sleep. He suffered an attack every night. The attacks always came at the same time—one at 9 PM and the other at 5 AM. The first attack seemed to be set off after eating or after considerable laughter.

When the problem became intolerable, Frederick S. was given *natrum sulph.,* and within half an hour the attack disappeared, and the family got its first complete night's sleep in ages. At the end of two months, the attacks had disappeared completely. In addition, the child, who had been withdrawn and underweight, became more outgoing, gained weight and took on a healthy color.

In another remarkable case, Ann M., a 23-year-old woman, moved to Cleveland from South Carolina. Small-boned, blonde and usually in excellent health, she began to suffer from asthma and a tight, short cough. This went on for two miserable years. After taking *natrum sulph.* in a high concentration, she recovered completely in just two weeks. She also experienced better all-around health.

No one knows why *natrum sulph.* is a good treatment in asthma cases, but doctors have reported case after case where it cured long-standing asthma completely. Perhaps this is due to its ability to attract twice its bulk in water-containing waste products and then remove this waste from the bloodstream. Or possibly the amazing results are related to its incredible ability to heal the mucous membranes. Whatever the reason, consider *natrum sulph.* your ally if you suffer from asthma.

It is possible that the powers of this amazing remedy are due to the fact that it is a "super" cell salt—that is, it works in the fluids *between* the cells, acting as part of the process that enables the cells to discern what they need in the fluids outside themselves and what substances are harmful and must be eliminated. *Natrum sulph.* acts as a "sensor" and has the ability to aid the cells in finding sustenance.

Natrum sulph. in Combination

Natrum sulph. is a good treatment alone as well as in combination. A biochemical "cocktail" of *natrum sulph.* and silica is a potent tonic for asthma attacks. The silica will help with the symptoms of the asthma, and the *natrum sulph.* gets right to the root of the malady. Many of the other cell salts will be helpful in specific kinds of asthma (check the Simplified Remedy Guide for these). *Natrum sulph.*, however, is the number one asthma remedy.

Just how powerful is it? One gentleman, Gene V., was promptly cured of his asthma attacks by taking *natrum sulph.* during one of his worst spells. His asthmatic breathing had been so pronounced that people could hear him coming from a great distance. Doctors had checked his lungs and found nothing unusual, but the attacks continued. During a particularly terrible attack, he took low potency doses of *natrum sulph.* After that, the problem improved until he needed only occasional doses. His asthmatic breathing was gone.

In another case, Christine K., a 32-year-old woman whose grandmother had died from asthma, and who had suffered from it herself since the age of four, received great relief from *natrum sulph.* and *medorrhinium,* a botanical homeopathic remedy. Christine recovered from the asthma, but her doctor was worried by her mental state. She had many fears—fears of disease, fire, pain, insanity, high places, flying, strangers, spiders, snakes, and other things, and above all she feared spending money foolishly.

She also left her family behind in Denver for days on end, which caused them great anxiety. On one of her rovings, she wound up in San Francisco, where she met a homeopathic doctor. He gave her a large dose of *medorrhinium,* which eliminated her confused wanderings. She returned to her family and subsequently enjoyed life much more.

Asthma that is aggravated by wet, warm weather is especially likely to be helped by *natrum sulph.* Helen B., who had an acute case of asthma only when the weather changed, was promptly relieved of her symptoms by taking *natrum sulph.* When the problem returned two years later, she was again given a large dose and she never had another attack.

Diabetes and Digestion

Diabetes is another disease which *natrum sulph.* has been successful in treating. Years ago, when insulin was discovered, everyone thought that diabetes was finished as a life-threatening disease. However, diabetics frequently develop fatal side effects, including cardiac failure. Some medical authorities believe that increased dietary intake of sugar is the cause of the dramatic increase in cases of diabetes.

Natrum sulph. can play an enormous role in treating many problems related to digestion, which is why it is sometimes an important treatment in diabetes. It has also been helpful to people with gallbladder troubles. Of course, if you have gallbladder problems, you should not treat yourself; see your doctor.

Influenza

Natrum sulph. was said to cure the flu by Dr. Charles S. Vaught, who added that excessive catarrh, itching, scabies or eczema are all signs of a sodium sulphate deficiency. Dr. Vaught himself was suffering from influenza in its earliest stages and "headed it off at the pass" by taking *natrum sulph.* Other doctors have reported curing difficult cases of influenza by using this remedy. When Bill A., a 26-year-old bookkeeper, went to work one day, he was feeling perfectly well. Then suddenly, at 10 AM, he became tired and weary. He began to sneeze and his temperature went up. These were all the signs of the flu. *Natrum sulph.,* taken every hour on the hour, enabled him to feel better immediately, and he returned to work the next day.

One authority on biochemistry suggests dissolving two or three tablets each of *ferrum phos., natrum sulph.,* and *kali mur.* in a glass of hot water and sipping it when influenza threatens. The doses, in the 6x potency, should be repeated every thirty minutes.

Head Injuries

An interesting characteristic of *natrum phos.* is its ability to help in cases of head injuries. In this era of busy freeways and city streets, we can easily be involved in accidents having long-lasting effects.

In one case, Bob R., a second-year medical student, was in a motorcycle accident and suffered severe head trauma, as well as fractures of several ribs and vertebrae. He remained in a coma and was fed intravenously for several months. Finally, his doctors decided to perform a very delicate operation to save him. Ten days after the operation, there seemed to be no hope. Then one doctor suggested *natrum sulph.* in the 200x potency.

Within a week after the patient started this treatment, a dramatic improvement began. In just three weeks the patient was conscious. He could eat, write simple words, converse in a whisper, and read and understand newspapers and magazines. The hospital where this occurred has since ordered *natrum sulph.* to be administered in all such cases.

Other Benefits

Natrum sulph. cell salts largely control the action of the liver according to biochemical theory. During a spell of humid, oppressive weather, a few doses of this cell salt will help you to recover from that sluggish, run-down feeling.

A deficiency in *natrum sulph.* can result in a number of psychological symptoms. Irritability, often a symptom of our fast-paced modern life, is the foremost indication of this. *Natrum sulph.* will yield fast, comforting results, provided that the short temper you have is due to a sodium sulphate deficiency rather than just irritating in-laws or overdue bills.

Natrum sulph. is a natural sleeping potion. If you have trouble falling asleep and have restless dreams, if your sleep is unrefreshing, if you find yourself waking too early or too frequently, then a dose of *natrum sulph.* every hour, beginning a few hours before bedtime, will do what the prescription medicines promise. Moreover, this cell salt remedy is completely harmless. There is no way that you can become addicted to it. When you have taken it for a very short period of time, you will discover that your sleep-related problems will disappear, giving you the refreshed appearance and peace of mind that come with improved sleep.

Also, if you find yourself getting cold in bed at night, especially in the hands or lower limbs, consider *natrum sulph.* your natural electric blanket.

Feelings of discouragement are another indication that you may need *natrum sulph.* Most people have a hard time getting started in the morning. However, if you always feel depressed and despondent in the morning, think of *natrum sulph.*, which, if taken regularly as prescribed here, will bring you a much brighter mental outlook.

Natrum sulph. is also often helpful in cases of gout, and in alleviating pain connected with teeth and dentistry. Many illnesses for which this remedy is indicated really call for all three of the biochemical sodium remedies: *natrum mur.*, *natrum sulph.*, and *natrum phos.* You are advised to take a combination of these three cell salts if you are irritable due to biliousness, if you have a headache centered in the top of your head, if you suffer from dizziness, if you suffer from drowsiness, or if you have anxious dreams or nightmares.

Cell Salts
for
Youth and Beauty

For centuries, women have exchanged beauty secrets on how to develop and maintain glowing, vital loveliness at any age. Try this simple beauty plan involving cell salts and a minimal amount of effort for a period of thirty to sixty days, and you will be delighted with the results.

The Importance of Good Nutrition

As you have discovered, the twelve cell salt remedies can play a big part in restoring the health you may have lost as a result of a poor diet. The same poor diet that contributes to many health problems can also affect a person's appearance. Some of the indications that your body is not getting proper nutrition include a sallow complexion, incipient wrinkles and lines, poor muscle tone, general tiredness, dark circles under the eyes, insomnia, and dry skin. These problems detract from your good looks and can discourage you from even trying to look your best. But neglecting your appearance just causes more problems, and a vicious cycle is created.

If you are like lots of other women, you probably drag yourself out of bed in the morning, late for work or in a rush to get your husband and children off to work and school. You do not have time to fix yourself a good breakfast, even if you might prepare one for your family. So what do you give yourself? Black coffee and white toast. When your body is trying to tell you that it needs nutrition the most, to help you face the day squarely, it is ignored.

When noon rolls around, you probably find that you're absolutely starving. If you are at work, you raid the catering truck or vending machines and wind up with a lunch of dubious value—possibly a stale sandwich consisting of some processed cheese, ham and lettuce on white bread, more coffee, and a processed dessert. There are a lot of calories in this meal, but your body will be getting few of the nutrients it really needs for health and beauty.

At dinnertime, you are probably tired and not really up to preparing a nutritious meal. Fast foods or take-out are probably all you can manage. If this sounds at all like you, stop right now and consider this grim fact. If you continue neglecting and abusing yourself this way, all you can expect is an early old age. This is especially true if you are a young woman who feels that she has to starve herself all of the time to maintain a fashionably lean silhouette.

As you begin to plan a better nutritional program for yourself, the cell salt *calc. phos.* will help you. Take it before or after each meal. And then think about those meals. (Reread the section on *calc. phos.* on page 49, which will help you visualize your body's nutritional mechanisms at work.) You should avoid heavy, fat-laden meals. Get into the habit of eating a good breakfast. It can be as simple as a whole-grain cereal with a little fresh fruit and milk, or some fresh cheese, whole-grain toast, and fruit juice. Whole-grain cereals are extremely important in the diet for the precious vitamins and minerals they contain.

You can take your lunch with you to work. It should include a fresh, preferably raw, vegetable or salad, cooked eggs or cold meat, and maybe whole grain bread and butter. Avoid all soft drinks including those with artificial sweeteners. Drink at least eight glasses of pure water each day. Dinner should be the lightest meal of the day. A light soup or salad and some fruit is ideal.

Remember that sugar is absolutely useless in the diet. It serves no purpose nutritionally, and there are many health experts who believe that it can seriously damage your health. It also adds many empty calories. Bear in mind that it is an ingredient in many packaged foods. It is a good idea to read package labels carefully and substitute fresh fruits and vegetables for packaged or frozen fruits and vegetables. But beware of some so-called "natural" products. If you look closely at their ingredients, you may find that chemical preservatives or sugar are included.

To take cell salts and then eat sugar is like going to an Alcoholics Anonymous meeting and then going home and drinking a cocktail. Health is the result of a combination of things, of which the cell salts are an integral part. But the cell salts cannot work if you abuse your body in other ways.

Once your diet has become healthy, you will notice the beginning of a new you. You will lose unwanted pounds, have more energy, discover a brighter personality, and start looking better.

The Role of Cell Salts

Calc. phos. is the nutritional remedy that will make you feel good all over. It is routinely prescribed for sluggish, run-down conditions. It can help you regain your energy. *Kali sulph.* and *ferrum phos.* are also essential for any new health regimen. *Kali sulph.* and *ferrum phos.* both carry oxygen through your body and help restore your health. Try taking these remedies each day before you exercise.

Your exercise program need not be the regimented program you may have suffered through in school. An easy, personalized exercise program can be a wonderful tension reliever. It can quickly eliminate that sluggish, run-down feeling.

If you do not enjoy sports or working out in a gym, take a long walk or a hike in the most beautiful surroundings you can find. If you want to think things out, take your walk by yourself. If you prefer company, which may help pass the miles more pleasantly, invite your family or friends to walk with you. On a hot day, try a cool swim instead. If you feel exuberant, take advantage of your feeling by running for a while. You will soon discover that exercise has become something you associate with happy times. Each day, you will feel better immediately when you realize that it is the time of day to make yourself feel better by exercising.

135

At night, just before retiring, take *ferrum phos., kali sulph., mag. phos.,* and *natrum phos.* These will help you sleep well. Along with a healthy diet and exercise, your cell salt beauty plan should include plenty of sleep.

Getting enough sleep for your health might sound deceptively simple. Everybody knows that sleep is important, but how many people actually get enough sleep every night? Probably very few. If you cannot get to sleep until 3:30 AM because of insomnia and have to get up at 7:00 AM, you are not going to feel good. If you are one of the bleary-eyed souls who whiles away the wee hours of the night watching television because you cannot unwind any other way, try taking the above named cell salts. That way you will get your "beauty sleep."

Remember that part of being beautiful lies in having regular health habits—good diet, exercise, and enough rest. Erratic living does not help your appearance, and it does not prolong youth, either. A serene outlook on life and a sense of humor can also help you to develop both inner and outer loveliness.

Ferrum phos. is everyone's "beauty tonic." It is used in combination with other cell salts to treat many ailments, but it is also extremely effective by itself. It is also sometimes a good idea to take *kali phos.,* the soother of jangled nerves, to restore your peace of mind, promote a more positive attitude, and bring color back to your cheeks.

Ferrum phos. plays an important role in maintaining good health, which, of course, is the largest part of being beautiful. It is especially effective if your spirits are depressed, which will show on your face. All of the cell salt phosphates will help lift your spirits, but *ferrum phos.* will give you the physical basis for good health. If you are feeling discouraged, take *ferrum phos.* twice a day, morning and evening, and watch your gloomy symptoms disappear.

For Beautiful Hair and Nails

If you envy women with long, shiny hair and long, graceful fingernails, you are not alone. But you may feel that lovely hair and nails are an impossible dream. Commercial fingernail strengtheners may work at first, but they contain harsh chemicals. Hair conditioners are unreliable and full of strange chemicals. So what do you do? You take silica.

Silica, nature's cell cleanser, is recommended for many ailments. But it is especially useful for building up hair and nails. Take silica three times a day, morning, noon, and evening. At the same time, be sure that you are eating well and getting plenty of rest. Within thirty days, you should see your hair take on a healthy shine and split ends disappear. Your fingernails will be stronger, longer, and less inclined to break and split.

Eliminating Water Retention

Another problem that can detract from beauty is water retention. Many women who experience this find it to be worst just before their menstrual period, although in susceptible women it is sometimes an ever-present condition.

If you have a water retention problem, take *natrum sulph.* and *natrum mur.* before meals to help regulate your body fluids. You should also stop adding salt to the food you eat. A low salt intake will benefit your heart and may even protect you from some forms of cancer.

Since *natrum sulph.* and *natrum mur.* work to eliminate bloating and water retention, they will help you produce a sleek new body. Some of the other salts you are taking in this program will also help you prevent obesity. Try *calc. fluor.*—it holds off obesity and is also good for the enamel of your teeth.

By the way, if you are especially troubled by water retention before your period, try stepping up your exercise program. Exercise also helps relieve menstrual cramps, which are sometimes associated with water retention.

Eliminate Varicose Veins

Varicose veins are unattractive reminders that we are getting older. They are also painful. *Calc. fluor.,* the cell salt which promotes suppleness and elasticity, has been recommended for treating varicose veins for years along with *ferrum phos.* and silica, which you should be taking already.

To treat varicose veins, take *calc. fluor., ferrum phos.,* and silica in the morning and evening, but give them time to work, especially if you have had the condition for a long time. You should obtain comfort, relief, and improved appearance within a reasonable time. If you do not, or if the condition worsens, see your doctor. There are other medical procedures besides taking cell salts for this condition.

A Clear, Fresh Complexion

Silica, which you should already be taking for your hair and nails, is also good for your complexion. But another salt is especially helpful for your complexion—*calc. sulph.,* a healer and purifier of the blood. If your face tends to break out, it is best to take *calc. sulph.* before the pimples start discharging pus. If they have already started to discharge pus, take *kali mur.* in addition. The cell salts should be taken every two hours until the pimples have discharged the pus. Then take the cell salts only twice a day, morning and evening. You might have to take the cell salts every time your skin starts to break out again. Both *calc. phos.* and *kali sulph.* help build new skin cells, but you should already be taking these anyway. Also, for general skin health, stay away from greasy foods and too much salt and sugar.

Natural Cell Salt Cosmetic

Avocado is one of the best cosmetics you can buy. You can create your own avocado cosmetics, or you can buy avocado creams at health food stores. Do not be fooled by products from large chemical cosmetic firms that use a dab of avocado for sales appeal. These products are still essentially chemical and may be irritating or even dangerous.

To create your own avocado cream, puree avocado flesh and refrigerate it for three days. Then add one tablespoon of a multiple cell salts combination, dissolved in water and wheat germ oil, to the puree (or a health food store cream). The result will be a product that should help remove flabby jaw lines, sagging muscles, and crepe necks if it is used with consistency.

Why the avocado–cell salt mixture? Because avocados are nature's best emollient. They are rich in cell salts and natural humectant—a substance which draws water to itself. Water (not oil) creates soft, beautiful skin, and avocado applied to the skin, with cell salts and vitamin E (in the form of wheat germ oil) added, is just about the best cosmetic there is. Use it in your cell salt beauty plan. Use the avocado–cell salt cream on your face at night, and start using the cell salts conscientiously in your diet.

Other Beauty Problems

For acne, hair and scalp problems, obesity, warts, heavy perspiration, sunburn, fatigue, and premature aging, check the Simplified Remedy Guide for appropriate treatments.

Glossary

Acute. In cell salt terminology, "acute" indicates a particular health problem that appears suddenly or worsens. (See *Chronic*.)

Allopathy. Medicine other than homeopathic medicine—the practice of conventional medicine.

Biochemistry. Dr. Schuessler's simplified system of homeopathic medicine. Dr. Schuessler believed that the twelve cell salt (or biochemical) remedies contain all of the active ingredients of the large homeopathic *materia medica*. (See *Homeopathy*.)

Chronic. A health problem or ailment that has existed for a relatively long period without any noticeable change in symptoms or modalities. In cell salt terminology, the opposite of acute.

Constitutional remedy. The particular cell salt remedy that you may need, sometimes regardless of symptoms. However, the symptoms you display generally indicate which remedy is your constitutional remedy.

Holistic medicine. Biochemistry is essentially holistic in nature; that is, it treats the entire individual, not merely his or her symptoms or illness. Each person is considered different from everyone else, with his or her own particular requirements for health. Holistic medicine is involved in all phases of health—diet, environment, and mental state as well as disease.

Homeopathy. The system of medicine founded by Samuel Hahnemann in the eighteenth century. Homeopathy focuses on two concepts: like cures like, and small doses are the most effective. An example of the former is the vaccination, whereby a person is given a shot of a particular disease virus to stimulate his or her own resistance to the disease. Dr. Schuessler's system, biochemistry, is a simplified version of homeopathy.

Materia medica. The thousands of mineral and botanical remedies used as homeopathic medicines, of which the twelve cell salts are simplified versions.

Osmosis. The process by which the cell salts get to the cells that specifically require them. This involves seepage through the cell membrane and eventual penetration into the cell.

Potency. The dosage of a particular cell salt. For example, the 6x potency contains far less than one part per million of active ingredient. The rest of the tablet is made up of milk sugar. In the cell salt system, the less active ingredient there is in the tablet, the higher the potency is, in accordance with homeopathic theory.

Provings. Symptoms of ill health produced in a healthy person by a homeopathic or biochemical remedy. According to the theory of "like cures like," the remedy should then improve the health of a person suffering from the same symptoms.

Suppuration. Pus, or the release of pus.

Synergist. A chemical or mineral that works with another chemical or mineral to perform a particular task. In the cell salt system, many of the cell salts, especially those in the same mineral group, work together to achieve a particular result.

Trituration. The process whereby the ingredient in a particular cell salt is broken down into minute doses according to homeopathic theory.

Resource List

Where to Obtain Cell Salts

Most health food stores and many regular drug stores now carry the individual cell salts and combination formulas. Look for them in the nutritional supplement section.

You can also order cell salts online and over the phone through such companies as Homeopathy Overnight, which offers cell salts from three major manufacturers: Dolisos, Standard Homeopathic, and Boericke and Tafel. For more information, go to their website, www.homeopathyovernight.com, or call 1-800-276-4223.

Many people prefer to deal directly with the cell salt manufacturer. Generally, prices range around $6.00 per 100 tablets. Different companies have different policies for shipping costs and minimum orders. All the firms mentioned here have toll-free order numbers, and many also have websites, so it's easy to check with them about details.

Boericke and Tafel, Inc.
2381 Circadian Way
Santa Rosa, CA 95407
1-800-876-9505

Boericke and Tafel, Inc., manufactures the individual cell salts in various potencies. It does not offer a combination remedy.

Boiron-Bornemann, Inc.
Box 449
6 Campus Avenue
Building A
Newtown Square, PA 19073
Consumer information center:
1-800-BOIRON1 (264-7661)
1-800-BLU-TUBE (258-8823)
98c West Cochran Street
Simi Valley, CA 93065
1-800-258-8823

Boiron sells the individual cell salts in 6x and 30x potencies, in tablet and pellet form. (Homeopathic remedies operate more quickly in pellet form.) It also offers Biophosphates, a combination of some of the cell salts, specifically designed for treating general intellectual and physical fatigue. Additionally, the firm offers a combination of all twelve of the cell salts.

Dolisos America, Inc.
3014 Rigel Avenue
Las Vegas, NV 89102
1-800-365-4767
www.lyghtforce.com/Dolisos/

Dolisos is one of the more established homeopathic manufacturers. It offers cell salts in 6x and a variety of other potencies, both in tablet and pellet form. Additionally, it offers a twelve-salt combination.

Luyties Pharmacal
4200 Laclede Street
St. Louis, MO 63108
1-800-HOMEOPATHY

Luyties is another long-time homeopathic manufacturer. It offers all the cell salts individually; no combination remedies.

Newton Homeopathic Laboratories, Inc.
2360 Rockaway Industrial Boulevard
Conyers, GA 30207
1-800-448-7256
Info line: 1-800-NOSODE 3

Newton sells the individual cell salts, although it offers only 10x and 15x potencies, in tablet and liquid form. It does not manufacture any combination remedies.

Standard Homeopathic Company

P.O. Box 61067
204-210 West 131st Street
Los Angeles, CA 90061
1-800-624-9659

Standard Homeopathic is the best-known manufacturer of cell salts. The firm has been manufacturing homeopathic remedies since 1903. It offers the cell salts in the traditional 3x and 6x potencies as well as in 12x and 30x. It offers several combination remedies including Bioplasma, a twelve-salt supplement designed to be taken daily.

Washington Homeopathic Products, Inc.

4914 Del Ray Avenue
Bethesda, MD 20814
1-800-336-1695 (Orders Only)
1-800-556-0738 (Pet and
  Equine Orders)

Washington Homeopathic offers single remedies in 6x and 12x potencies, as well as a combination of all twelve.

Index

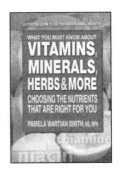
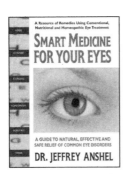